The Russian Medical Humanities

The Russian Medical Humanities

Past, Present, and Future

Edited by Konstantin Starikov
and Melissa L. Miller

LEXINGTON BOOKS
Lanham • Boulder • New York • London

The text of chapter 5, "Pauline Tarnowsky and the Russian Influence on Cesare Lombroso's *Criminal Woman*," was previously published in Russian by New Literary Observer Publishing House in 2020 and is published here in English by permission.

Published by Lexington Books
An imprint of The Rowman & Littlefield Publishing Group, Inc.
4501 Forbes Boulevard, Suite 200, Lanham, Maryland 20706
www.rowman.com

86-90 Paul Street, London EC2A 4NE

British Library Cataloguing in Publication Information Available

Library of Congress Cataloging-in-Publication Data

Names: Miller, Melissa Blair, 1972– editor. | Starikov, Konstantin, editor.

Title: The Russian medical humanities : past, present, and future / edited by Melissa Miller and Konstantin Starikov.
Description: Lanham : Lexington Books, [2021] | Includes bibliographical references and index.
Identifiers: LCCN 2021030782 (print) | LCCN 2021030783 (ebook) | ISBN 9781498592154 (cloth) | ISBN 9781498592161 (ebook)
Subjects: LCSH: Medicine and the humanities—Russia. | Medical ethics—Russia.
Classification: LCC R702 .R87 2021 (print) | LCC R702 (ebook) | DDC 174.20947—dc23
LC record available at https://lccn.loc.gov/2021030782
LC ebook record available at https://lccn.loc.gov/2021030783

Contents

Table and Figures

TABLE

FIGURES

Acknowledgments

We owe a debt of gratitude to the many people who have made this volume possible. We would like to thank our contributors, whose incisive work and cheerful collaborative spirit have brought this book to fruition. We are especially grateful to Natalia Vygovskaia for her help and expertise in preparing the research for this collection. At Lexington Books, Eric Kuntzman, Alexandra Rallo, and Kasey Bedun have been a joy to work with. This project benefitted from a Summer Residency Fellowship from the National Humanities Center and from research support from the Summer Research Lab at the University of Illinois at Urbana–Champaign. In particular, the insight and dedication of Lynn Miller, Brooke Andrade, and Joe Lenkart and their teams have been invaluable.

Introduction

Konstantin Starikov and Melissa L. Miller

In May 2014, Samara State Medical University hosted a conference on "Humanitarian Engagement as Innovative Practice in Biology and Medicine."[1] The term "humanitarian engagement" in the conference's title, according to E. I. Burlina, one of many distinguished faculty and organizers of the event, was a self-conscious attempt to address issues in the medical humanities through the interdisciplinary connectivity of the humanities and biomedicine. The international scope of the conference also suggested that Russian colleagues may have become more receptive to the field of "medical humanities," a term which has not been fully accepted yet in the Russian language. In the title of her subsequent article, which highlights the results and accomplishments of the conference, Burlina uses the calqued term "meditsinskaia gumanitaristika." Nevertheless, the calqued term is not sufficient; it needs to be placed in the Russian context. As Burlina elaborates, "But what to call the area of study that focuses on how humanitarian engagement is related to the ways in which medicine functions in society? In the West the term 'Medical Humanities' is used. But in Russian, as journalist and doctor Marina Pavlova justly notes, a translation of this concept has not yet been conceived of, except for the unwieldy 'humanitarian sciences connected to medicine.'"[2] The takeaway points of this short article may be that Russian philosophers of medicine and faculty at medical programs throughout Russia, just like at Samara, have been actively working in the field of medical humanities without attempting to introduce the term until quite recently.

If the term "medical humanities" has not been widely used in Russia and the search for relevant literature on the topic of medical humanities in library catalogs and databases requires other search strategies and keywords, it is our proposition that the field of Russian medical humanities exists, and the interdisciplinary activities under the umbrella of Russian medical humanities in and outside of the Russian Federation deserves a closer examination. As of today, the practice of Russian medical humanities, as we argue, is fragmented into subjects that cover a wide range across a network of international interdisciplinary communities. The interdisciplinary nature of medical humanities that includes subjects as philosophy (including ethics), anthropology, law, psychology, history, religious studies, literature, and the arts is an intrinsic characteristic of medical humanities as an emerging academic field, but also as a mixture of practical methods in medical professionalism. In our view, the richness of the cultural impact of Russian medical humanities and the expertise of scholars in the field of Russian studies and of Russian medical educators has not been fully tapped into by medical practitioners and educators in the West. Indeed, in the field's excellent first textbook in English, titled *Medical Humanities: An Introduction*, the authors admit that they are limited by their own knowledge of only English and German, and invite readers to share their own perspectives on texts and cultures outside of America and Western Europe.[3] Similarly, one may also argue that the conceptualization of "medical humanities" as a twentieth-century social experiment in reforming medical education in the West is gaining momentum in Russia in hope of reimagining traditional Russian medicine's ethical identity.

The medical humanities traverse national boundaries. Both in North America and Europe, as well as in Russia, many medical schools expose students to the humanities as they relate to medicine and bioethics. The degree of depth and range of the subjects offered may vary, as do formal and informal educational models, from integrated modules and structured lectures to elective courses, workshops, or extracurricular club activities. There are also master's programs in which public health and medical anthropology play an important role in promoting medical humanities topics to medical students who otherwise would not encounter them in their courses. One could argue that the history of medicine and philosophy is more likely to be accepted as useful in medical schools across cultures. Since modern Russian medicine is based on the European model, it is also noteworthy that some old traditions in Western medical education, such as the study of Latin or German that disappeared in the West, continue to thrive in Russian medical education.

The formalization of medical humanities as an academic discipline has been gradually introduced across the world, including Russia. The trend to "re-humanize" medical practice in the United States in the 1960s and 1970s began as a desire to bridge the divergence of the humanities and science in postmodern society. On both sides of the Atlantic there was a development of discourse communities in which dilemmas of medical professionalism led to a critical view of the commercialization of medicine and the replacement of traditional ethical commitments of healthcare practitioners. The technological advancements and technical disciplines of the second half of the twentieth century only exacerbated the pessimistic worldview of critical thinkers who had been warning of the moral and ethical perils of science and technology as self-absorbing worldviews incapable of making space for the humanities. The concept of "crisis" therefore is to be found in the articulation of the necessity of engagement with humanistic traditions as a common trope in the social contexts of Western free-market societies and the post-Soviet realities of the practice of medicine in Russia.

In post-Soviet Russia, the sense of "crisis" was two-fold. As Irina Siluyanova, head of the Department of Biomedical Ethics at the Pirogov Russian National Research Medical University in Moscow, argues in her book *Bioethics in Russia: Values and Laws*,[4] the democratization of Russian society in the 1990s led to the adoption of the rather recent tradition of bioethics which had emerged in the United States during the 1960s and 1970s, the decades of social instability due to racial tensions, the Vietnam War, and the women's rights movement. Similarly, the socio-economic instability of the 1990s in Russia coincided with the rethinking of the Soviet medical profession as an ideological paradigm. "Democratization in Russia," Siluyanova explains, "from a cultural point of view, became a fundamental prerequisite for the remarkably intensive development of bioethics that has taken place in our country. In recent years we have witnessed the growth of information networks that allow for the continued expansion of this knowledge, both in the areas of scientific research and education, as well as in the popular and academic spheres."[5]

The 1990s spurred a wave of structural reorganizations in Russian medical education. For example, in 1995, the Department of Humanities and Bioethics was created at St. Petersburg State Pediatric Medical University with the express purpose of expanding the cultural and medical worldviews of future doctors. The nurturing of moral values such as the humane treatment of both "healthy and ill people, based on respect for the uniqueness and value of every living being" is taught by exposing students to Russian history, philosophy, and the history of medicine.[6] Beginning in 1997 the Department also introduced the subjects of economics, jurisprudence, and bioethics. In 1991, the Volgograd State Medical University reorganized its department, which had been founded in 1974, as the Department of History and Cultural Studies, with a focus mainly on Russian history and general cultural history. Today, one of the topics taught and researched in the Department is the "Humanization of Medical Education." These two examples illustrate an evolution typical of many Russian medical, scientific, and educational institutions in which departments that for decades taught the philosophy of Marxism-Leninism were either reformed or split up into new departments with a moral reorientation toward Western, liberal, and pre-1917 Russian philosophical principles. The culmination of this trend was the year 2000, the symbolic end of the twentieth century and beginning of the new twenty-first century. In the year 2000, bioethics became a federal standard in Russian medical education as part of the requirements for becoming a medical professional.[7]

The integration of bioethics into Russian medical education did not mean that the critical debates surrounding euthanasia, abortion, organ donation, patient confidentiality, and a myriad of other ethical issues solved the socio-economic problems of the post-Soviet medical profession, such as corruption, commercialism, and the detachment of oneself from social or political activism. With the fall of the Soviet Union, Russian society entered a period of economic uncertainty which only aggravated public health issues such as poor life expectancy and an increase in cases of preventable diseases among the adult population. Not paid enough by the state-run health system, Russian doctors, especially those working in the provinces, have been traditionally working in conditions of financial instability, even as the healthcare system has been undergoing a major reform since 2010.

The role of medical humanities in Russian medical education is important in emphasizing doctor-patient relationships in the current social, political, and economic conditions of modern Russia. Teaching humanities to medical students or engaging doctors to practice medical humanities in complex, and often demoralizing, professional work environments would imply that an integrative approach to medicine as a scientific and humanistic field of human knowledge is prioritized over the current paradigm in which histories of medicine, philosophy, psychology, anthropology, bioethics, foreign languages, and, to a lesser extent, literature, music, and the arts are being taught as academic disciplines or sources of intellectual information without an opportunity to discuss, understand, and conceptualize oneself as an individual in the process of one's own moral development. Recent trends in medical education in Russia and the Former Soviet Union reflect a growing preference for such an integrative model, and not just in the traditional centers of culture and politics, such as Moscow, St. Petersburg, and Kiev. For example, the official press at the Arkhangelsk State Medical Academy has published their own reader titled *Medicine in the Works of Russian Writers: An Anthology for Medical Students*.[8] This collection of short stories, longer prose pieces, and informative essays is readily available on the Internet, and its stated purpose is to allow medical students all across the Russian Federation to learn about the best practices of patient care from a wide variety of creative works by Russian authors.[9] Likewise, the Academic Senate at Kharkiv National Medical University in Kharkiv, Ukraine, which provides instruction in both Russian and English languages, recommends that medical students and current physicians study medical ethics and deontology by analyzing literary texts from their lengthy official list. This resource, *Medicine Through the Mirror of World Literature: An Annotated Bibliography*, consists of both classic and contemporary creative works and is also available for download as a free PDF from the University.

A medical practitioner who does not work in Russia or a medical student who is not interested in spending some time in Russia may wonder: what good is it to learn about Russian medical humanities? We believe that the practical purpose and the increasingly theoretical rationalization of promoting the field of medical humanities globally is to underline the humanness of all individuals across cultures. Our healthcare systems may be different, our economic and political systems may be incompatible, even our social values may be at odds with each other at various periods in history. Whether we like it or not, the trends of globalization in science and technological advancements in the twenty-first century will bring us in closer proximity than ever before to other humans, animals, and the natural environment we all inhabit. Since the humanities help us to interpret ambiguities, to hone critical thinking skills, and to experience the "other" from a non-standard point of view, a closer look into the Russian worldview of medical humanities is valuable not only as an intellectual exercise, but also, and more importantly, because it provides empathetic insight into the experience of medical encounters which all cultures grapple with. Therefore, we anticipate that this volume will prove useful not only to current and future health practicioners, but also to a broader audience of readers who are seeking to make compassionate and informed decisions about healthcare for their loved ones and for themselves.

Although the title of our book may dissatisfy an English-speaking reader in search of a comprehensive history of Russian medical humanities, the editors of this volume have chosen it deliberately, aspiring to show that the ongoing work of many scholars, educators, and medical professionals can be brought together in a diverse community of Russian medical humanists. As editors, we have invited a small number of contributors to begin conversations about the field of medical humanities by sharing their own research and topics of interest. The main theme that runs through this book is one that emphasizes the contribution of Russian medical humanities to the past and present aspirations of humanity as a whole: the betterment of human society beyond borders. In many ways, transnational collaboration in the Russian medical humanities is just beginning, and as a result, there are important facets of this research, such as disability studies, film and media studies, and folk medicine, that we were unable to include. Each of these areas deserves its own separate study in order to do justice to the material. It is our hope that we will be able to incorporate this vital work in a future volume.

The present collection consists of nine chapters, which range in tone and style between academic research and personal observations, close readings of literary texts, and surveys of professional activities, fact, and opinion. This volume of essays also places in close proximity voices from the Russian Federation and the United States. In this connection, our book is divided into two sections. Part I, "History and Education," explores past and present humanistic trends in Russian medical training, while part II, "Medical Encounters in Literature and Culture," examines how Russian authors and cultural figures, some physician-writers, some without professional background in medicine of any kind, have positioned healthy and ailing bodies in their creative work. We can proudly say that in addition to the interdisciplinary nature of this volume, it is also international in scope, for the first section features the following scholars whose work is based in Russia: Evgeniya L. Panova is Professor in the History of Medicine Department at Sechenov University; Maria S. Tutorskaya is Head of the Methodical Cabinet at the Center of the Development of the Medical Museums in Russia, Moscow State University of Medicine and Dentistry; Maria P. Kuzybaeva is a historian and independent scholar with a specialty in medical museum studies; Jonathan McFarland is Director of the Academic Writing Office at Sechenov University; and Irina Markovina is Head of Foreign Languages, also at Sechenov University in Moscow.

Panova and Tutorskaya place the concept of charity in the center of the development of the medical profession in Moscow. They show how the medical community in the Russian Empire evolved into an independent economic force capable of using medical care and medical education as a tool for social reforms. With the focus on the historical contributions of faculty from Moscow University, Tutorskaya and Panova offer a detailed analysis of grassroots initiatives to reform medical education in the context of the Russian state's centralized system of governance. We hope that the reader will take away from the chapter the optimistic message that charity as an essential aspect of medical humanities is a valuable tool for future doctors' social activism.

As a former curator of the Medical Museum at the Russian Academy of Medical Sciences (1995–2000), Kuzybaeva explores in her chapter issues that underscore the importance of preserving anatomical collections in the twenty-first century. In a brief exposition of the history of Russian anatomical and pathologic-anatomical collections, Kuzybaeva overviews the state of the historical collections based on the examples of three major centers of medical education in the Russian Empire: the Imperial Moscow University, the Imperial Kazan University, and the Imperial Medical Surgical Academy. She is especially interested in the history of formation and maintenance of the osteological collections. As a genuinely concerned medical humanist, Kuzybaeva attempts to convince her reader that negative trends of disregard for the preservation of anatomical and pathologic-anatomical collections in Russia can be rectified by raising awareness of the contributions these collections have made to the medical education of students and the general public.

McFarland and Markovina's chapter demonstrates the value of an interdisciplinary, intercultural, and international approach to engaging future doctors at Sechenov University and outside its walls, literally across the world. Therein they describe their "Doctor as a Humanist" initiative, an ongoing medical humanities project with an innovative approach in Russian medical education. McFarland and Markovina reflect on their own experience and the experience of their students who actively engage in the exploration of humanistic principles in the medical profession. The focus of the chapter is on the reporting of goals, strategies, and accomplishments, which captures not only the temporal dimension of described events, such as conferences and symposia, but also, and most importantly, emphasizes the continuity of the Russian humanistic tradition in medical education at Sechenov University. After all, Anton Pavlovich Chekhov, the great Russian writer and internationally acclaimed playwright, studied the art of medicine at the same university (then Moscow University Faculty of Medicine). Today, just like Chekhov's characters may fluently speak in English on the stages of London and New York, medical students at Sechenov University discuss articles from *BMJ* and reflect on classic texts in medical humanities in English, such as Oliver Sacks' *A Leg to Stand On* and William Styron's *Darkness Visible: A Memoir of Madness*.

In his report of survey results from 2017, Starikov offers a critical analysis of Slavic faculty awareness, attitudes, and practices regarding the teaching of medical humanities. The objective of the survey was to collect data and, based on the interpretation of findings, to challenge Slavic scholars to enhance professional and humanistic teaching of Russian literature in medical education. Starikov raises the questions of educational competencies, pedagogical techniques, and the benefits of co-teaching among Slavic scholars and medical staff of Chekhov's short stories in order to strengthen the humanistic education of medical students in North American medical schools.

The second half of the volume is devoted to Russian cultural figures and their creative explorations of doctors and patients, as well as to the complex negotiations that characterize their relationships to each other. White's chapter focuses on the pioneering work of Russian female physician Praskov'ia Tarnovskaia, arguing convincingly that her studies of female criminals, such as prostitutes and thieves, actually served as a formative influence on what has long been considered the groundbreaking work in this field in the West, Cesare Lombroso and Guglielmo Ferrero's *Criminal Woman, the Prostitute and the Normal Woman*. In so doing, White not only establishes Tarnovskaia's importance for medical studies in the West, but he also demonstrates that the personal case histories that went along with the female offenders' official files have contributed to the lasting interest in Tarnovskaia's research in criminal anthropology.

Similarly, Miller's essay also seeks to bridge the divide between the medical humanities as it is conceptualized in the United States and how they have traditionally been practiced in Russia. Drawing upon recent research on narrative medicine in the Anglophone tradition, which holds that treating patients as authors of their own individual stories will lead to better health outcomes and is championed by such leaders in the medical humanities in the West as Rita Charon and Sayantani DasGupta, Miller's essay argues that narrative medicine has also animated the careers of famous Russian physician-writers as well, such as Anton Chekhov and Mikhail Bulgakov. Taking Bulgakov's short-story cycle *A Country Doctor's Notebook* as her focal point, Miller demonstrates how Bulgakov's creative work, written right after the Russian Revolution of 1917, actually prefigured both the advantages and the challenges posed by contemporary notions of narrative medicine. In so doing, Miller argues that Russian literature of the past can yield valuable insights into medical training and patient care in the present.

By contrast to many of the chapters in this section, Vygovskaia's contribution explores the work of a Russian physician-writer who is little known in the English-speaking world, Vikentii Veresaev (pseudonym of Vikentii Smidovich). In her treatment of his novel *The Deadlock*, set during the Russian Civil War, Vygovskaia argues for the uniqueness of Veresaev's perspective on these historic events. Due to his dual professional roles as both doctor and writer, Veresaev was able to present the conflict between the Reds and the Whites as a complex dialogue, rather than portraying this time period as an epic battle between good and evil. Vygovskaia demonstrates how Veresaev creates a diagnostic narrative that chronicles the ways in which the disease of violence threatens the health and wellbeing of those on both sides of the cataclysm.

Brintlinger's essay focuses on Russian literature's tradition of setting stories in the medicalized space of the ward in order to comment on society as a whole. She examines ward fiction from two important Russian doctor-writers and two writer-patients—Anton Chekhov, Maxim Osipov, Alexander Solzhenitsyn, and Julia Voznesenskaya—in order to evaluate the efficacy of potential treatment interventions. While these male writers, as Brintlinger notes, "seem to feel compelled to 'diagnose' not just their characters, but the society they live in," Voznesenskaya's text *Women's Decameron* (1986) challenges this archetype. Constructed as a set of one hundred stories narrated by ten women in a Soviet maternity ward, *Women's Decameron* grants narrative agency to her characters, as well as a respite of mutual understanding in an environment that is chaotic and often cruel. As Brintlinger shows, Voznesenskaya's work posits a female version of the traditionally powerful male gaze, flipping the roles so that women patients take charge of their own meaning.

Finally, Gheith's essay combines her professional backgrounds both as a professor of Russian culture and as a hospice social worker in order to examine the profound ways in which Russian literature can help us work with patients and their families. Drawing on her experience as an educator, Gheith showcases how Russian literature is useful in teaching the medical humanities. Her article is a case study, showing her hospice work with dementia patients and how contemporary Russian author Liudmila Ulitskaia's *The Kukotsky Case* can help to deepen our understanding of patient and family dynamics. The article also explores how patients and families are related to aspects of the Russian work, and how it helped family members reconcile with the disease and have greater compassion for the patients and for themselves.

As Anne Hudson Jones, a pioneer in the field of medical humanities in the US, notes in her authoritative article "Why Teach Literature and Medicine? Answers from Three Decades," the trajectories of programs in medical humanities in other countries and cultures deserve their own investigations.[10] By examining various aspects of humanities-focused medical education and training, as well as questions surrounding health and healthcare, illness and recovery in the Russian literary and cultural tradition, both abroad and in the United States, this volume seeks to fill some of this gap. Such work is especially important for the post-Soviet context, as readers and writers alike have expressed frustration at the ways in which Russian culture has traditionally approached discussions concerning the body. Author Liudmila Ulitskaia, whose fiction Gheith analyzes in her essay in this volume, treats themes that were "more or less forbidden in Soviet lit: eroticism, sexual minorities, abortion, alcoholism, the disabled, diseases, and of course, death."[11] When readers have asked Ulitskaia whether or not she considers herself a pioneer for addressing such taboo topics out in the open, she laments that while "it never occurred to [her] to use any filters,"[12] the Russian language is also very "chaste," because "all we have are medical terms, the unusable dirty words, not included in any academic dictionaries, or euphemisms. Writing about delicate, very intimate experiences with such philological resources is a challenge."[13] At the same time, the very themes listed above—as well as a viable language to discuss them in—also prove essential for the modern medical humanities. It is our hope that the articles in this volume will serve as a catalyst for further conversations about the nature of embodiment in Russian literature and culture. As befits the multifaceted and interdisciplinary nature of the medical humanities themselves, our contributors fulfill a wide variety of professional roles, from literary scholars, educators, translators, and poets to medical historians, librarians, museum curators, and social workers. It is our hope that the chapters to follow will spark new insights into what it means to understand another's pain, to heal, and ultimately, to be human.

NOTES

1. The original title of this conference in Russian is "Gumanitarnoe obespechenie innovatsionnoi deiatel'nosti v biologii i meditsine." All translations in the introduction are ours unless otherwise noted. The website for the conference may be found here: http://www.samsmu.ru/events/2014/200514/. Last accessed January 26, 2020.

2. Burlina, E. Ia., "Paradigmy meditsinskoi gumanitaristiki. Mezhdunarodnaia mezhdistsiplinarnaia konferentsiia 'Gumanitarnoe obespechenie innovatsionnoi deiatel'nosti v biologii i meditsine,'" *Izvestiia Samarskogo nauchnogo tsentra Rossiiskoi akademii nauk*, t. 16, No.2(2), 2014: 267–269; 268.

3. Cole, Thomas R., Nathan S. Carlin, and Ronald A. Carson, *Medical Humanities: An Introduction,* New York: Cambridge University Press, 2015, 11.

4. The original title of this book in Russian is *Bioetika v Rossii. Tsennosti i zakony*. This groundbreaking work was the first textbook in Russian for undergraduate and graduate students, as well as physicians, that was devoted to problems of professional ethics in medicine in the context of the Russian moral and ethical tradition.

5. Siluyanova, Irina, *Bioetika v Rossii. Tsennosti i zakony*, Moscow: Grant, 2001, 42–43.

6. "Istoriia kafedry gumanitarnykh distsiplin i bioetiki," Sankt-Peterburgskii gosudarstvennyi pediatricheskii meditsinskii universitet, accessed January 6, 2020, https://gpmu.org/university/structure/departments/gumanitar/history_human.

7. Siluyanova, *Bioetika v Rossii*, 43.

8. The original Russian title is *Meditsina v proizvedeniiakh russkikh pisatelei: Khrestomatiia dlia studentov meditsinskikh uchebnykh zavedenii*. Compiled by A.Kh. Satretdinova. Astrakhan: Izd-vo GOU VPO AGMA, 2009.

9. The original title in Russian is *Meditsina v zerkale mirovoi literature: annotirovannyi bibliographicheskii ukazatel'*. Compiled by I.V. Kirichok, V.M. Serpukhova, O.V. Ozerkina. Edited by I.V. Kirichok. Kharkov: KhNMU, 2014.

10. Jones, Anne Hudson, "Why Teach Literature and Medicine? Answers from Three Decades," in *New Directions in Literature and Medicine Studies*, Stephanie M. Hilder, ed., London: Palgrave-Macmillan, 2017. 31–48; 41–42.

11. Ulitskaya, Lyudmila, "Ludmila Ulitskaya," in *Contemporary Russian Fiction: A Short List; Russian Authors Interviewed by Kristina Rotkirch*, translated by Charles Rougle, edited by Anna Ljunggren and Kristina Rotkirch, 174–192. Moscow: Glas, 2008, 181.

12. Ulitskaya, "Ludmila Ulitskaya," 181.

13. Ulitskaya, "Ludmila Ulitskaya," 179–180.

WORKS CITED

Burlina, E. Ia. "Paradigmy meditsinskoi gumanitaristiki. Mezhdunarodnaia mezhdistsiplinarnaia konferentsiia 'Gumanitarnoe obespechenie innovatsionnoi deiatel'nosti v biologii I meditsine.'" *Izvestiia Samarskogo nauchnogo tsentra Rossiiskoi akademii nauk*, t. 16, No.2(2), 2014: 267–269.

Cole, Thomas R., Nathan S. Carlin, and Ronald A. Carson, *Medical Humanities: An Introduction.* New York: Cambridge University Press, 2015.

"Istoriia kafedry gumanitarnykh distsiplin i bioetiki." Sankt-Peterburgskii gosudarstvennyi pediatricheskii meditsinskii universitet, accessed January 6, 2020, https://gpmu.org/university/structure/departments/gumanitar/history_human.

Jones, Anne Hudson. "Why Teach Literature and Medicine? Answers from Three Decades." In *New Directions in Literature and Medicine Studies.* Stephanie M. Hilder, ed. London: Palgrave-Macmillan, 2017. 31–48.

Meditsina v proizvedeniiakh russkikh pisatelei: Khrestomatiia dlia studentov meditsinskikh uchebnykh zavedenii. Compiled by A.Kh. Satretdinova. Astrakhan: Izd-vo GOU VPO AGMA, 2009.

Meditsina v zerkale mirovoi literature: annotirovannyi bibliographicheskii ukazatel'. Compiled by I.V. Kirichok, V.M. Serpukhova, O.V. Ozerkina. Edited by I.V. Kirichok. Kharkov: KhNMU, 2014.

Siluyanova, Irina. *Bioetika v Rossii. Tsennosti i zakony*. Moscow: Grant, 2001.

Ulitskaya, Lyudmila. "Ludmila Ulitskaya." In *Contemporary Russian Fiction: A Short List; Russian Authors Interviewed by Kristina Rotkirch*, translated by Charles Rougle, edited by Anna Ljunggren and Kristina Rotkirch, 174–192. Moscow: Glas, 2008.

Part I

HISTORY AND EDUCATION

Chapter One

Physicians' Charity as a Lynchpin in Forming Medical Community

Evgeniya L. Panova and Maria S. Tutorskaya

In this chapter we analyze historical aspects of physicians' charity, defined as generosity and helpfulness especially toward the needy or suffering,[1] in the Russian Empire in general, as well as individual stories of medical professionals and institutions that donated money, were involved in fundraising for medical care, and provided charity care for those who needed it. We focus on the second part of the nineteenth century: in addition to being known as *La Belle Époque* or the Golden Age of Russian medicine, we also consider this period after the Great Reforms and before the Revolution of 1905 to be the time of medical professionalization in Russia.[2]

In this chapter we focus on personalities and cases related to the Medical Faculty of Moscow University for several reasons. First, Moscow University had the largest enrollment of any medical school in the Russian Empire. Most Russian physicians studied in Moscow and were thus influenced by the professors and their mindset. In the 1890s the Clinic Campus on the Devichye pole (Maidens' Field) in Moscow became a model for the construction of the clinical complexes at Kazan and Kharkov Universities. Secondly, people used to call Moscow the "benefactor" and the "All-Russian poorhouse." Moscow was more comparable to other large Russian cities than the capital St. Petersburg in terms of the forms of charity available, as well as in terms of the structure of the various charitable organizations.[3] In this way the Moscow public charity experience formed the basis for other cities.

Traditionally, secular medicine and charity were the domain of the Russian state. Tsars, emperors, and their familiars invited foreign doctors of medicine to Russia and donated money to the poor. Charity became an ongoing governmental activity, not only a church affair, during the reign of Peter I in the early eighteenth century. The state established the first public charity institutions, including hospitals, poorhouses, and welfare establishments, and started formulating a regulative body to administer care for the needy. During the eighteenth century, emperors and empresses encouraged wealthy people to follow their lead and donate money. For example, Catherine II commanded that funds which had been earmarked for the construction of a monument in her honor instead be given to charitable institutions. She said that instead of receiving offerings she wished "to erect a monument in the hearts of my subjects, rather than in marble."[4]

By the beginning of the nineteenth century the charity regulations for accepting donations were clearly defined. The Act of January 4, 1816, determined both "the non-acceptance of donations from vicious people," as well as the "absence of an award to them for these [donations]."[5] This Act proclaimed that only persons respected by their fellow citizens for their integrity and piety could participate in charity. At the same time, there was a place for personal initiative and the emergence of new types of charity. In this connection it is worth mentioning two vivid individual examples: Dr. Fedor Haass (1780–1853) and Nikolai Pirogov (1810–1881). Dr. Haass is known as the "holy doctor of Moscow."[6] He was the "town physician" of Moscow, deeply engaged in prisoners' healthcare and founded a hospital for the homeless sick. Nikolai Pirogov was a military surgeon who first used anesthesia in the form of ether on the battlefield. He was one of the most influential doctors in Russia, both during his lifetime and after his death, even becoming the subject of a famous Russian Christmas story by the writer Alexander Kuprin (1870–1938) titled "A Wonderful Doctor."

The criteria regarding who could and who should be engaged in charity were developing not only in Russia during the first part of the nineteenth century. According to the Code of Medical Ethics published by the American Medical Association in 1847, "physicians were encouraged, as a duty to the public, to provide limited, gratuitous services to the poor."[7] Physicians' work in hospitals included the "delivery of health care to the public and in the academic and clinical training of physicians,"[8] but these charity activities were "incorporated into the gentlemanly ethic of noblesse oblige."[9] Similarly, the philanthropic intentions of the medical community were not the definitive feature of Russian medicine at that time, but rather, they have their own particular characteristics related to the specific historical aspects of charity and medical practice in the Russian Empire.

The beginning of the organization of medical care in Russia is usually attributed to the turn of the sixteenth and seventeenth centuries, when the state decided to create the Pharmaceutical Ministry, a single body that was responsible for providing medical care to the tsar and his family.[10] Foreign professionals were invited to work at this institution as doctors, pharmacists, and surgeons. The management of the Pharmaceutical Ministry was entrusted to a select group of Russian nobles or boyars, who were among those closest to the tsar. For example, one of its first leaders was the future tsar Boris Godunov.[11]

During the seventeenth century, known as the Time of Troubles, the Russian army was involved in numerous armed conflicts, such as the Russo-Polish and Russo-Swedish Wars, as well as the suppression of several riots. Soldiers who suffered during war or captivity could submit a petition to the tsar asking for mercy and treatment. There are several examples of this kind documented in the Pharmaceutical Ministry's archive. Sagittarius Andrei filed a petition in 1648 about treating his son: "my son got a spinal fracture when his sledge overturned in Arzamas. Besides yours, the sovereign's, physicians and doctors, there is no one who can heal. Merciful sovereign, Tsar and Grand Duke, Alexey Mikhailovich . . . please, order your sovereign healers to treat my son. Tsar, sovereign, have mercy."[12] In 1661, Ivan Vasilyevich Samarin, who had returned from captivity, asked for treatment of wounds received in battle: "Your servant, Ivashka Vasilyev, son of Samarin, presses your forehead . . . favor for your serf for my service and for my total dedication, treat my wound with your sovereign doctor . . . Tsar, sovereign, have mercy."[13] As these examples demonstrate, during the seventeenth century scientific (European) medical treatment was subject to the mercy and charity of the tsar.

In the seventeenth century and the first half of the eighteenth century the main role in the development and organization of medical care and medical education belonged to foreign medical specialists. They also taught in the first medical school in Russia, which opened under the auspicies of the Pharmaceutical Ministry in 1654. Petr Vasilyevich Postnikov (1666–1702), having graduated from the University of Padua in 1694, became the first Russian to receive the diploma of Doctor of Philosophy and Medicine. However, due to the lack of European-educated diplomats in Russia at that time, P.V. Postnikov was forced to devote his career to diplomacy, rather than to medicine. The Hospital School, founded in 1707 in Moscow by Nikolai Bidloo (1674–1734), Peter the Great's Dutch physician, became the first educational institution in Russia that systematically trained medical specialists. Graduates of this and other hospital schools (in St. Petersburg, Kronstadt, etc.) were intended exclusively for military medical service.

Thus, when the Imperial Moscow University, henceforth called Moscow University, was founded in 1755, and its medical faculty was established in 1758, most physicians in Russia were foreigners. However, neither this relatively small number of foreign doctors, nor the hospital schools (later reorganized into military medical academies) could provide the amount of medical professionals that the Russian state required. Unlike graduates of medical and surgical academies, who were sent to military service immediately after graduation, students who graduated from the Medical Faculty of Moscow University had much more freedom to manage their professional careers. The best graduates continued their studies abroad and, after returning to Russia, they became the leaders of scientific schools and departments at their alma mater, medical-surgical academies, and the universities established in the early nineteenth century, such as in Kazan, Vilnius, Kharkov, etc. Among them are: M.Ya. Mudrov (1776–1831), A.I. Auver (1804–1864/1865), and G.A. Zakharin (1829–1898) in the field of therapy; and N.I. Pirogov (1810–1881), F.I. Inozemtsev (1802–1869), and I.N. Novatsky (1825–1902) in the field of surgery. These and other outstanding doctors and teachers not only founded Russian medicine, but also contributed to the formation of the professional community of Russian physicians.

The emergence of an independent professional medical community in Russia, capable of being a significant social force, began in the second half of the nineteenth century. The first and most obvious reason for its appearance was the substantial growth in the number of students at institutes of higher medical education during the nineteenth century and, consequently, the number of certified Russian-speaking doctors. For example, if in the 1813/1814 academic year, 30 students were studying at the Medical Faculty of Moscow University, then in 1855 it was already 817.[14] In addition, by the beginning of the 1880s, the number of students had almost doubled compared with the 1860s.[15] In 1857, Russian Emperor Alexander I drew attention to the growing number of medical students. He ordered the Ministry of Public Education to find out whether the conditions at universities corresponded to the increased academic load and to take the necessary measures for the proper organization of the educational process. However, no action was taken at that time.

Additionally, the possibility for graduates of medical faculties of universities to engage in private medical practice or work in private medical institutions led to an increase in physicians' material wellbeing and allowed some of them to achieve financial independence. However, it would be fair to say that this was particularly true for the most respected university professors who had been able to achieve outstanding results in medical science and teaching. Those physicians who were less lucky in their career were themselves targeted as the objects of charity. Due to the high risks of disease and trauma in their work and the absence of any type of social insurance or social assistance from the state, physicians were forced to organize mutual self-help funds.

For example, in his novel *The Death of Ivan Ilyich*, Leo Tolstoy describes the most fashionable and expensive Moscow doctor of that time, G.A. Zakharin (1829–1898). Zakharin, an outstanding Russian therapist and teacher whose students founded therapeutic, gynecological, and pediatric clinical schools, was also known for his wealth. A significant part of it was acquired not through his private practice, though he sometimes did receive thousands of rubles for one visit, but instead through joint financial ventures with his friends who were bankers, many of whom were also his patients.[16] Zakharin generously donated considerable amounts of these funds to help needy medical students. In 1880 he provided 10 thousand rubles for scholarships at the medical faculty of Moscow University, and also contributed 2 thousand rubles for the issuance of lump-sum benefits.

The growth in the number of Russian-speaking doctors, along with their increasing authority and levels of financial well being, led to the emergence of a large number of medical societies. The onset of these professional organizations was, in a way, a consequence of Russia's defeat in the Crimean War. Numerous deaths due to mass infections, the short supply of medical dressings and drugs, and poor management of military medical support indicated the necessity of new forms of interaction between medical professionals and state officials. Specialized and regional societies were established in rapid succession. Doctors sought increased authority and autonomy. In order to gain a voice in public discourse in Russia, they created professional journals and published bulletins of their societies' meetings. By the end of the century there was a number of specialized regular all-Russian medical congresses. In 1897 the 12th International Medical Congress took place in Moscow and St. Petersburg.

As a result of these advances, medical charity emerged as a special type of social (philanthropic) activity. Its role in the development of the professional medical community in Russia, in our opinion, is underestimated. What began as an internal assistance program quickly took on much greater significance. The heyday of medical charity in Russia occurred during the last quarter of the nineteenth century. We consider the creation of the Clinical Campus on Devichye Pole by Moscow University's professors to be one of the best examples of physicians' charity in Russia. Their investments in the project included not only providing their own money and expertise, but also running a successful fundraising campaign and sacrificing opportunities to maintain lucrative private practices of their own.

As we have already noted, by the end of the 1850s the increase in the number of students of medical faculties at Russian universities had become so serious that it attracted the attention of the Emperor. By that time, the medical faculty of Moscow University had been experiencing a severe shortage of training facilities and laboratories: the number of clinical disciplines had increased and new theoretical departments had been organized. All this required special facilities for teaching and scientific research. Most acutely, there was a severe lack of clinical teaching facilities: by the beginning of the 1860s, clinical teaching at Moscow University was conducted in the clinic at Rozhdestvenka and at the New Catherine Hospital. The clinic on Rozhdestvenka was a facility of Moscow University where students practiced the basic skills of patient care. The clinic was divided into two departments: therapeutic and surgical. The New Catherine Hospital served as a clinic for Moscow University, where students mastered complex skills in the fields of therapy and surgery. The total bed capacity of these clinics was 370 beds. This was not enough to cover the needs of medical students' training at that time. The situation was further complicated by the fact that the buildings at the disposal of the Faculty of Medicine were dilapidated and needed major repairs.

Moscow University Professor of Medicine A.I. Polunin (1820–1888) was the first who brought this problem to the attention of the public. In his article "Considerations on the Measures That Can be Taken to Ensure That at Imperial Moscow University the Number of Professors of the Medical Faculty and Teaching Assistants Corresponds to the Exorbitant Number of Medical Students," published in the *Moskovskie vedomosti* newspaper on January 15, 1861, he described the deplorable state of teaching in the university's clinics. There, he wrote,

> Students should look after every patient. Each student should see how the professor examines the patient, and everyone should examine the patient himself. But 100 or 200 students cannot fit in a hospital ward. Naturally, with such a large number of students, only a few students who are prompt and diligent can examine the patients along with the professor; the others are jostling in the corridors and arrive at the hospital room after the professor has approached the patient. How to train such a number of students in the diagnosis of diseases of the lungs or the heart? Can this huge number of students see the operations that the professor performs? Can they follow the treatment of wounds, bandaging them after surgery? How to teach so many students practical obstetrics? Is it possible to train 200 students in one obstetrics clinic? Obviously, the enormous number of students makes teaching difficult and severely hinders learning.[17]

The situation was complicated by the introduction in 1863 of the General Statute of Universities, which decreed that universities must start teaching new clinical disciplines, such as urology, pediatrics, and gynecology, as well as nervous and skin diseases.[18] Also, the Charter established new theoretical departments which required that special facilities for teaching and scientific research must be organized. The medical faculty of Moscow University had to create these new clinical and theoretical units using their own materials and technical resources. In 1866 the Departments of Pediatrics (with 11 beds) and Urology were organized at the Clinic at Rozhdestvenka. Three years later at the Therapeutic Clinic, located at the New Catherine Hospital, a Department of Nervous Diseases (with 20 beds) and a ward for patients with skin diseases (with 6 beds) were opened. In 1873 and 1874, at the expense of the Therapeutic Clinic, 16 beds were allocated for teaching general diagnostics and therapy and a gynecological ward with 4 beds was organized. These innovations, on the one hand, allowed faculty to begin teaching special sections of clinical medicine at Moscow University, however, on the other hand, the creation of specialized units naturally led to a decrease in the number of beds in faculty and hospital clinics, a reduction in educational and auxiliary facilities, the crowding of patients in wards, and finally to the deterioration of teaching and patient care conditions.

This is how V.K. Rot (1848–1916), a follower of Alexei Yakovlevich (A.Y.) Kozhevnikov (1836–1902), the first head of the Department of Nervous Diseases and the founder of the Moscow Neurological School, described the teaching conditions in the Department, opened in 1869:

> Having become an associate professor, A.Y. [Kozhevnikov] lectured under very adverse conditions for a long time: there were no teaching assistants and no funds were given for them; there were no drawings or anatomical specimens; it was not possible to demonstrate on patients during a systematic course of nervous diseases and psychiatry, which was being conducted in another part of the city, far from the clinic for nervous diseases. . . . For the clinic for nervous diseases, 20 beds were allocated to the New Catherine Hospital, and that was it: all other needs related to teaching, research, the treatment of patients, scientific studies, etc. . . . A.Y. had to satisfy. Clinical lectures were given in wards, there were no lecture rooms, and the clinical classes during A.Y.'s first years of teaching were successful only due to the limited number of courses and the division of students who attended the clinic for one semester into two parts: students received 1–2 patients each, visited them daily, carefully wrote medical records and kept diaries. But soon the number of students increased to 200, once even to 313 per course. Not a single ward could accommodate half of the students, lectures were carried into the corridor, where only the first rows of students could see and hear anything, while the majority of them were actually deprived of the opportunity to get something out of the lecture.[19]

Thus, by the beginning of the 1870s, the problem of organizing and conducting daily operations at the medical faculty of Moscow University had become even more fraught.

In November 1872, the chief physician at the New Catherine Hospital and professor of the Hospital Surgical Clinic N.I. Novatsky submitted a plan outlining the expansion of Moscow University's clinics to the Medical Faculty. He offered to sell the land and the building of the Faculty Clinic at Rozhdestvenka (which was located in the very center of Moscow), which would yield about 1 million rubles in silver. An additional sum of 150 or 200 thousand rubles in capital was needed, which could be provided by the Hospital for Laborers, which at that time did not have its own building. Combining these two sums, it would be possible to build a clinic with 1,000 beds. As Novatsky proposed, it could accommodate the Hospital for Laborers managed by Moscow University, which would also become their clinical base. Although the Medical Faculty had approved Novakovsky's project, the University Council rejected it without offering an alternative.

Since it had become apparent that the government was either unable or unwilling to address the shortages of material and technical resources plaguing the Medical Faculty, Moscow University's professors were forced to seek funding on their own. Since the initiatives of Polunin and Novatsky did not meet with official approval from above, the doctors and teachers of the Medical Faculty had only one option: to launch active fundraising efforts to attract benefactors to the project. Soon the first results appeared. In 1882 E.V. Paskhalova donated 140 thousand rubles for the construction of the Obstetrics Clinic for 40 beds. Professor of the Obstetrics Clinic A.M. Makeev recalled:

> Initially, E.V. Paskhalova had a desire to help in relieving the suffering of several women during childbirth, with the best possible help. The inconvenience and cramped conditions of our clinic gave us the idea of directing Ms. Paskhalova's good will towards the establishment of a new Obstetrics Clinic, where women in labor could receive the most up-to-date medical care. Our proposal was gladly accepted by the donor, and the idea of building a new Obstetrics Clinic at the existing Faculty Clinics became possible.[20]

A few months later, Professor A.Y. Kozhevnikov managed to convince Countess V.A. Morozova to donate 450 thousand rubles for the construction of a Psychiatric Clinic for 60 beds in honor of her husband.[21] V.A. Morozova became one of the main benefactors of the construction of the Campus on Devichye Pole, having added to this donation a plot of land of 13 thousand square sazhens, where the Psychiatric (1887) and Neurological (1890) Clinics were later built. V.K. Rot, using the example of A.Y. Kozhevnikov, described the various organizational activities that were deployed by professors of Moscow University to promote the project:

> The project was grandiose; its implementation, except for the University, depended on many factors. In order to achieve the desired result, it was necessary not only to defend the project, but also to evoke active sympathy for it, highlighting its importance with bright colors, outlining its expediency with very impressive arguments, and thoroughly and effectively grouped data. A.Y. was born to perform this task, and, of course, he deserves the main part of the credit for the successful outcome of the case.[22]

The donations from E.V. Paskhalova and V.A. Morozova had prepared the groundwork for soliciting generous donations from Moscow merchants, many of which, as we assume, were organized with the direct participation of Moscow University's professors, primarily by the dean of the Faculty of Medicine N.V. Sklifosovsky. In addition to the Obstetrics (1889) and Psychiatric Clinics (1888), which were funded with the money of E.V. Paskhalova and V.A. Morozova, private donations were used to construct the following facilities: the Gynecological Clinic (1889) with 40 beds was made possible by a gift from T.S. Morozova; the Pediatric Clinic (1891) with 25 beds was funded by M.A. Khludov; the Clinic of Skin and Venereal Diseases (1895) was built with funds from G.G. Solodovnikov; the General Outpatient Clinic was funded by V.A. Alekseev; a Gynecological Institute with a clinic (1896) for 25 beds was made possible by a donation from P.G. Shelaputin; and with the financial assistance of Bazanova, an Ear, Nose, and Throat Clinic was built. The total amount of private donations for the construction and equipment of the Clinical Campus on the Devichye Pole is not definitively known. According to the most conservative estimates, the amount of private donations is not less than a third of the total cost of the design, construction and equipment of the entire Clinical Campus.

Private donations became "a mute reproach to the university administration and the government, which was unable and unwilling to solve this important issue in time."[23] It was the financial investments of E.V. Paskhalova and V.A. Morozova that pushed the Medical Faculty to return to the discussion of the project first presented by Professor Novatsky in 1873.[24] However, many of Novatsky's principal provisions were later revised. At the beginning of 1883 a commission of the Medical Faculty was established under the chairmanship of N.V. Sklifosovsky. Professors of the Medical Faculty invariably participated in all the meetings and commissions held by the University Council, the Trustee of the Moscow Educational District, and the Minister of Public Education, in order to resolve issues related to the construction of the Clinical Campus on the Devichye Pole. The Faculty Commission proposed that the University Board apply to the Moscow Duma for a plot of land on the Devichye Pole. In the autumn of 1884, the Moscow Duma "decided to cede to the University's full ownership, a plot of land on the Devichye Pole belonging to the city, spanning 40 thousand square sazhens."[25] The next step was to draw up the architectural plans for the Clinical Campus. The Faculty Commission unequivocally stated that professors of the Medical Faculty involved in the work of the commission would take the lead in drafting the project. During the whole year of 1885 preparations were carried out by the Faculty Commission together with the architect K.M. Bykovskii.

According to experts, the decision to involve professors in planning the Clinical Campus predetermined the success of the project.[26] Each specialist presented his recommendations on construction, based on the specific features of each building as a specialized medical, educational, and scientific institution. Proposals from prominent hygienist F.F. Erisman allowed for the creation of an exemplary system of sanitary facilities that provided both water supply and wastewater disposal for the buildings of the Clinical Campus, as well as a ventilation and heating system in the clinics and institutes. The recommendations of the professors N.V. Sklifosovsky (1836–1904), V.F. Snegirev (1847–1917), and A.M. Makeev (1829–1913) became decisive in the design and construction of the Surgical, Gynecological, and Obstetrics Clinics. A.Y. Kozhevnikov designed both the Psychiatric and the Neuropathological Clinics. In addition, he managed to secure permanent state funding for the Psychiatric Clinic. As V.K. Rot recalled,

> A.Y. had to work out a plan for a new psychiatric clinic. He went to Kazan to get acquainted with the construction of the new district hospital, examined the Psychiatric Clinic in Leipzig during his trip to Karlsbad in 1883, involved people from whom he hoped to get practical instructions, studied the economic considerations, made a detailed estimate of expenses for the maintenance of the clinic, and got the annual amount of 30 thousand rubles to fund the project from the State Treasury.[27]

In July 1887, the Emperor Alexander III approved the project and a budget of 2.15 million rubles for the construction of the Clinical Campus. The University was obliged to transfer the land and the building of the Clinic on Rozhdestvenka Street to the Ministry of Finance. The sum allocated by the State Treasury was 875 thousand rubles less than the estimate drawn up by the Technical and Construction Committee of the Ministry of Internal Affairs. As F.F. Erisman noted, the Trustee of the Moscow educational district P.A. Kapnist applied for an increase in the loan for the construction up to 3,025 thousand rubles; however, the Minister of Education,

> quite agreeing that the above-mentioned amount is necessary for the execution of the project, nevertheless, did not dare to ask the State Council to increase the loan up to 3,025 thousand rubles, and at the same time, regarding the previous demand for a loan of 2150 thousand rubles, asked for a reduction in construction by 875 thousand rubles. The lack of funds might be made up for by the treasury, donations or from other sources, and then buildings that had been temporarily excluded would be constructed as necessary for the University.[28]

Thus, the funds allocated by the State Council for the construction of the Clinical Campus on Devichye Pole were not enough to finance the entire project. However, the Clinical Complex was fully built and equipped by 1897. Apart from the auxiliary subdivisions, it consisted of 13 buildings, which housed 15 clinical institutions with 710 beds and 6 scientific and educational institutes. It is not known where the deficient funds came from. We assume that the problem of finding the necessary financial resources was solved by the professors of the Medical Faculty both at the beginning and at the end of construction.

This long and loud campaign alerted the state authorities to the necessity of the transformation of teaching and support facilities at universities. In 1888, Emperor Alexander III approved a large-scale state project for the construction of the clinical complexes at Kazan and Kharkov Universities. As in the case of the construction of the Clinical Campus on Devichye Pole, professors of Kazan and Kharkov Universities played a significant role in the creation of these clinical complexes.[29] Thus, the joint work of the professors in organizing the construction of the Clinical Campuses in Moscow, Kazan, and Kharkov shows that by the end of the nineteenth century in Russia the foundation was laid for a stable and cohesive professional community of physicians, which became a serious force capable of solving global social issues with the involvement of the state and financial support of donors.

The successful completion of the construction of the Clinical Campus pushed the professors of the Medical Faculty of Moscow University to undertake new, socially important initiatives. Remarkable examples of physicians' charity in the Moscow Neuropathological School headed by A.Y. Kozhevnikov show that the founders of the University clinical schools inspired their students' active engagement in charitable campaigns, as well.

After the construction of the Psychiatric Clinic on Devichye Pole, the old Department of Nervous Diseases of the New Catherine Hospital continued its work. From 1892 to 1911, G.I. Rossolimo (1860–1928), as the head of the department, paid for all the necessary teaching assistants with his own funds.[30] Despite the huge role A.Y. Kozhevnikov played in the construction of the Psychiatric and Neurological Clinics, he decided not to stop there. Kozhevnikov's long-cherished dream was the construction of a Neurological Annex near the clinic where chronic diseases of the nervous system could be studied. For the construction and design of the Neurological Annex Kozhevnikov had to ask benefactors for financial contributions, as the university agreed to cover the costs of patient care only. Philanthropists donated 100 thousand rubles to the organization of the Annex, the most significant contribution of 50 thousand rubles coming from V.A. Morozova. "Sympathizing with the idea of such a shelter," wrote G. Pribytkov, a pupil of Kozhevnikov,

> V.A. Morozova expressed a desire to contribute 50 thousand rubles to the university for the construction and furnishing of the necessary building and, wishing that the shelter could be used mainly by poor people, she set the condition that 2/3 of the patients should be treated in the annex for free. To provide the rest of the funds [Kozhevnikov] had to resort again to people who sympathize

> with the project, despite the fact that the university took over part of the costs of patient care; fortunately, such persons were found, and he received donations of another 50 thousand rubles: from M.O. Morozova, 20 thousand rubles, E.V. Paskhalova, 25 thousand rubles, and Princess M.A. Shcherbatova, 5 thousand rubles. Thus, this idea of [Kozhevnikov's] was realized: the Annex was opened on October 10, 1891, where observation and treatment of patients is carried out as strictly scientifically as in the clinic, of which he is an integral part.[31]

Kozhevnikov's next goal was the creation of the Neurological Museum, which would contain anatomical specimens necessary for training. At the founding of the museum in 1892 Kozhevnikov contributed 3,000 rubles as the basic capital. Later he donated 10 thousand rubles for the updating of collections. In total, he donated about 16 thousand rubles for the maintenance of the museum.[32] After Kozhevnikov's death the Neurological Museum was renamed in his honor. The creation of the museum was the first step toward establishing the Research Neurological Institute. It was founded by the Moscow Society of Neuropathologists and Psychiatrists and mostly consisted of Kozhevnikov's followers after his death. For this purpose, the capital bequeathed by Kozhevnikov, as well as funds raised by the members of the society, were used. The whole amount consisted of about 76 thousand rubles.[33] The construction of the Neurological Institute was begun by V.K. Rot in 1909, when he was the head of the Clinic of Nervous Diseases after the death of his mentor. Construction was completed with the assistance of V.A. Muratov in 1913. Shortly before his death in 1916, V.K. Rot gave his microscope and 1,000 rubles to Muratov for the Neurological Institute.[34] In 1911–1917 G.I. Rossolimo founded the Institute of Pediatric Neurology and Psychology at his own expense, which was donated by its founder to Moscow University.[35]

CONCLUSION

Thus, we may state that after more than three centuries of the initial development of the medical profession in the Russian Empire, an independent medical community emerged in Russia in the last quarter of the nineteenth century. Using the example of the Medical Faculty of Moscow University's professors, we can follow the considerable work they spearheaded in the field of charity in order to solve difficult problems related to clinical teaching and treatment. In so doing the medical community[36] finally took shape, and medical professionals were able to get involved in solving social problems through active interaction with other social groups, such as state officials, merchants, architects, engineers, etc. These interactions were tightly connected with solving current problems in medical care. Doctors focused on the social causes of the diseases and considered medicine to be a social institution, while in turn, medical care was a social service and a social obligation. This approach depended both on the existence of a large number of medical professionals and on the strong credibility of these professionals in Russian society.

Growth of the enrollment at the medical faculties of the Universities was recognized by state officials, but how to increase the number and quality of clinical sites for the growing number of students became a matter for the medical professors of these educational institutions to solve. They took various steps to find solutions, such as investing their own money, seeking out generous sponsors among their patients and acquaintances, and advocating for higher education for women. Higher Women's Courses were established in St. Petersburg, where they were known as the Bestuzhev Courses, as well as in Moscow and other Russian cities. Funding for these institutions originated mostly from private donors, not from the government. The largest lump-sum contribution was made by the merchant M. Sibiryakov, who donated 50 thousand rubles. Beyond this, there were contributions made by medical professors, such as therapist S. P. Botkin (1832–1889), who donated 20 thousand rubles in his will. The hygienist A. P. Dobroslavin (1842–1889), the pathophysiologist V. V. Pashutin (1845–1901), the therapist V. M. Tarnovskii (1837–1906), and the microbiologist I. Mechnikov (1845–1916) lectured at these courses free of charge. Small amounts were contributed by peasants, students, and other people. Botkin's friend Ivan Sechenov (1829–1905), the author of *Reflexes of the Brain*, wrote, "The Bestuzhev Courses of the first period of their existence represent an edifying example of what a private initiative in Russia would look like if it were given open space to grow."[37] Sechenov lectured at the Bestuzhev Courses for years without receiving a salary. He later moved to Moscow and started to lecture at the Moscow Higher Women's Courses. Of this program, he wrote,

> The establishment had good intentions: to give an opportunity for teachers to receive further education and to educate women. It didn't cost the government anything, didn't require any rights for women students, and lived quietly for itself, unconnected to organized government supervision. Therefore it was closed as soon as the Guerrier Higher Courses were established. Self-government is not fashionable in Russia.[38]

In spite of the difficulties described by Sechenov, the professors of Moscow University managed to transform medical education in the oldest university in Russia, even considering the passive role of authority in this case. Such vigorous and effective educational initiatives on the part of these professors was only possible due to their understanding of the essential social origins of medicine. We believe that modern medical students should be taught according to these examples. That is why reducing the medical humanities in favor of clinical disciplines in medical schools' curriculum does not allow future physicians to comprehend the whole significance of the social role of medicine, and often even prevents them from participating in different forms of social activity, even in the cases when it is necessary for patients' treatment.

NOTES

1. *Merriam-Webster Dictionary*, s.v. "charity," accessed June 10, 2019, https://www.merriam-webster.com/dictionary/charity.

2. Frieden, Nancy Mandelker, *Russian Physicians in an Era of Reform and Revolution, 1856–1905*, Princeton: Princeton University Press, 1981.

3. Bogdanov, V.P., *The History of Charity in Russia, Moscow and the Moscow Press of the End of the XIX Century: A Textbook for Undergraduate and Graduate Programs,* Moscow: Yurayt, 2019, 7.

4. Ulyanova, G.N., "Charity in the Russian Empire from the End of the Eighteenth to the Beginning of the Twentieth Century," Dissertation. Moscow, 2006, 272.

5. *The Complete Collection of the Laws of the Russian Empire.* Collection I. T. XXXIII. No. 26061, January 4, 1816.

6. Vashkau, N.E., "The 'Holy Doctor' Fedor Petrovich Haaz," *The Bulletin of Volgograd State University*, Series 4: History, 2, (2012): 26–31, 26.

7. Kao, Audiey, "Physicians and the Obligation of Charity Care," *AMA Journal of Ethics* (2001). Web: https://journalofethics.ama-assn.org/article/physicians-and-obligation-charity-care/2001-06. Last accessed on December 29, 2019. No pagination.

8. Kao, "Physicians and the Obligation of Charity Care."

9. Kao, "Physicians and the Obligation of Charity Care."

10. In Russian, this entity is called "Aptekarsky Prikaz."

11. Mirsky, M.B., "The Origin of the Pharmaceutical Ministry," in *Essays on the History of Medicine in Russia (XVI–XVIII cent.)*, Vladikavkaz: Goskomizdat, 1995, 10.

12. Marchukova, S. M. *Medicine in the Mirror of History,* Saint Petersburg: European House, 2003, 241.

13. Marchukova, *Medicine in the Mirror of History*, 241.

14. Stochick, A.M. and S.N. Zatravkin, "On the Centenary of the Clinical Campus of Moscow University on Devichye Pole," *Problemy sotsialnoy gigieny, zdravookhranenia i istorii mediciny,* 6, 1997, 33–39, 33.

15. Stochick, A.M., "The History of the Creation of Moscow University's Clinical Campus on Devichye Pole. 100 Years of the Clinical Campus on Devichye Pole (1887–1997)." Paper presented at the Scientific-Methodological Conference of the Academy's Faculty, Moscow, 1997, 7.

16. Topolyansky, V.D., *Doctor Zakharyin: Legends and Reality. Anthology,* Moscow: Prava cheloveka, 2009, 530.

17. Stochick and Zatravkin, "On the Centenary of the Clinical Campus of Moscow University on Devichye Pole," 34.

18. The General Statute of Imperial Russian Universities, approved on June 18, 1863. In *General Statutes of Imperial Russian Universities of 1863 and 1884*. Odessa, 1901, 4–5.

19. Rot, V.K., *Aleksey Yakovlevich Kozhevnikov: An Obituary,* Moscow: Tipo-lit, I.N. Kushnerev and Co, 1902, 6.

20. Makeev, A.M., "The Obstetric Clinic Built by E.V. Paskhalova," in *New Clinics and Institutions (Clinical Campus) of Imperial Moscow University on Devichye Pole*, Moscow, 1891, 60.

21. Roeva, E.E., "The History of the Establishment of the Clinical Campus on Devichye Pole." Paper presented at the Scientific-Methodological Conference of the Academy's Faculty, Moscow: MMA named after I.M. Sechenov, 1997, 33.

22. Rot, *Aleksey Yakovlevich Kozhevnikov: An Obituary*, 18.

23. Stochick and Zatravkin, "On the Centenary of the Clinical Campus of Moscow University on Devichye Pole," 37.

24. Erisman, F.F., "A Brief History of the Construction of Moscow University's New Clinics," in *New Clinics and Institutions (Clinical Campus) of Imperial Moscow University on Devichye Pole*, Moscow, 1891, 2.

25. Erisman, "A Brief History of the Construction of Moscow University's New Clinics," 5.

26. Stochick and Zatravkin, "On the Centenary of the Clinical Campus of Moscow University on Devichye Pole," 38.

27. Rot, *Aleksey Yakovlevich Kozhevnikov: An Obituary*, 18.

28. Erisman, "A Brief History of the Construction of Moscow University's New Clinics," 5.

29. Bushueva, L., "The Professors Had to Undertake a Great Deal of Effort and Work to Construct the Clinic (The Creation of the New Clinics at Kazan University at the End of the 19th century)," *The Scientific and Documentary Journal Gasyrlar Avazy—The Echo of Centuries*, 1–2, 2012.

30. Bryleva, A.A. and E.L. Panova, "On the History of Clinical Neurology at Imperial Moscow University: The Department of Nervous Diseases at the New Catherine Hospital in 1911–1913," *History of Medicine,* Vol. 4. 4. (2017): 395–409, 397.

31. Pribytkov, G., *Aleksey Yakovlevich Kozhevnikov*, Moscow: t-vo tip. A.I. Mamontova, 1902, 3.

32. Central State Archive of the City of Moscow, F. 418. Op. 416. D. 67.

33. Lisitsyn, Y.P., *A.Ya. Kozhevnikov and the Moscow School of Neuropathologists*, Moscow: GIML Medgiz, 1961, 168.

34. Mikhaylenko, A.A., M.M. Odinak, and N.N. Yakhno, *The History of Russian Neurology: The Moscow Neurological School*, Saint Petersburg: SpetsLit, 2015, 158.

35. Lisitsyn, *A.Ya. Kozhevnikov and the Moscow School of Neuropathologists*, 250.

36. In Russian this term is "vrachebnoe soslovie."

37. Sechenov, I.M., *Autobiographical Notes,* Moscow: Scientific Word, 1907, 188.

38. Sechenov, *Autobiographical Notes*, 162.

WORKS CITED

Bogdanov, V.P. *The History of Charity in Russia, Moscow and the Moscow Press of the End of the XIX Century: A Textbook for Undergraduate and Graduate Programs.* Moscow: Yurayt, 2019.

Bryleva, A.A. and E.L. Panova. "On the History of Clinical Neurology at Imperial Moscow University: The Department of Nervous Diseases at the New Catherine Hospital in 1911–1913." *History of Medicine.* Vol. 4. 4. 2017. 395–409.

Bushueva, L. "The Professors Had to Undertake a Great Deal of Effort and Work to Construct the Clinic (The Creation of the New Clinics at Kazan University at the End of the 19th century)." *The Scientific and Documentary Journal Gasyrlar Avazy—The Echo of Centuries*. 1–2. 2012.

Central State Archive of the City of Moscow. F. 418. Op. 416. D. 67.

Erisman, F.F. "A Brief History of the Construction of Moscow University's New Clinics." In *New Clinics and Institutions (Clinical Campus) of Imperial Moscow University on Devichye Pole*. Moscow, 1891.

Frieden, Nancy Mandelker. *Russian Physicians in an Era of Reform and Revolution, 1856–1905*. Princeton: Princeton University Press, 1981.

Kao, Audiey. "Physicians and the Obligation of Charity Care." *AMA Journal of Ethics* (2001). Web: https://journalofethics.ama-assn.org/article/physicians-and-obligation-charity-care/2001-06. Last accessed on December 29, 2019. No pagination.

Lisitsyn, Y.P. *A.Ya. Kozhevnikov and the Moscow School of Neuropathologists*. Moscow: GIML Medgiz, 1961.

Makeev, A.M. "The Obstetric Clinic Built by E.V. Paskhalova." In *New Clinics and Institutions (Clinical Campus) of Imperial Moscow University on Devichye Pole*. Moscow, 1891.

Marchukova, S. M. *Medicine in the Mirror of History.* Saint Petersburg: European House, 2003.

Merriam-Webster Dictionary. https://www.merriam webster.com. Last accessed February 20, 2021.

Mikhaylenko, A.A., M.M. Odinak, and N.N. Yakhno. *The History of Russian Neurology: The Moscow Neurological School*. Saint Petersburg: SpetsLit, 2015.

Mirsky, M.B. "The Origin of the Pharmaceutical Ministry." In *Essays on the History of Medicine in Russia (XVI–XVIII cent.)*. Vladikavkaz: Goskomizdat, 1995.

Pribytkov, G. *Aleksey Yakovlevich Kozhevnikov*. Moscow: t-vo tip. A.I. Mamontova, 1902.

Roeva, E.E. "The History of the Establishment of the Clinical Campus on Devichye Pole." Paper presented at the Scientific-Methodological Conference of the Academy's Faculty. Moscow: MMA named after I.M. Sechenov, 1997.

Rot, V.K. *Aleksey Yakovlevich Kozhevnikov: An Obituary.* Moscow: Tipo-lit, I.N. Kushnerev and Co, 1902.

Sechenov, I.M. *Autobiographical Notes.* Moscow: Scientific Word, 1907.

Stochick, A.M. "The History of the Creation of Moscow University's Clinical Campus on Devichye Pole. 100 Years of the Clinical Campus on Devichye Pole

(1887–1997)." Paper presented at the Scientific-Methodological Conference of the Academy's Faculty. Moscow, 1997.

Stochick, A.M. and S.N. Zatravkin. "On the Centenary of the Clinical Campus of Moscow University on Devichye Pole." *Problemy sotsialnoy gigieny, zdravookhranenia i istorii mediciny,* 6, 1997. 33–39.

The Complete Collection of the Laws of the Russian Empire. Collection I. T. XXXIII. No. 26061. January 4, 1816.

The General Statute of Imperial Russian Universities, approved on June 18, 1863. In *General Statutes of Imperial Russian Universities of 1863 and 1884*. Odessa, 1901.

Topolyansky, V.D. *Doctor Zakharyin: Legends and Reality. Anthology.* Moscow: Prava cheloveka, 2009.

Ulyanova, G.N. "Charity in the Russian Empire from the End of the Eighteenth to the Beginning of the Twentieth Century." Dissertation. Moscow, 2006.

Vashkau, N.E. "The 'Holy Doctor' Fedor Petrovich Haaz." *The Bulletin of Volgograd State University*. Series 4: History, 2, (2012). 26–31.

Chapter Two

The History of the Formation and Maintenance of the Osteological Collections in Russia in the Nineteenth–Twenty-First Centuries

Maria P. Kuzybaeva
Translated from Russian by Konstantin Starikov

Today, Russian curators of anatomical collections share the worldwide concern about the long-term preservation of authentic bone remains and specialized collections, which are currently underutilized in the education of medical students. In Russia, declining conditions regarding the preservation of anatomical and pathologic-anatomical collections is not a new phenomenon. Challenges in maintenance have plagued these types of collections in Russia since their inception. In this brief article I will cover the basic history of the osteological collections in Russia and share specific examples from their evolution from the nineteenth to the first half of the twenty-first century.

The development of specialized scientific museums and collections in Russia began in the beginning of the nineteenth century. The foundations for such collections in the field of medicine were laid in the seventeenth and eighteenth centuries, thanks to the activities of the Apothecary Ministry (organized in the second half of the sixteenth century)[1] and the decrees of Tsars Alexei Mikhailovich and Peter I. Several academic museums were founded on the basis of the richest collections of the Kunstkammer, the first Russian museum, which was established by Peter I in Saint Petersburg in 1717 and completed in 1727. The purpose of these museums was to popularize scientific knowledge, to educate, and to disseminate the achievements of science in Russian society. This trend also manifested itself in the private collection of medical artifacts, which were part of the natural science collections of the Russian aristocracy and representatives of the medical profession. Medical educational institutions played an important role in the creation of museums and cabinets of curiosities, in which thematic collections, such as osteological collections, were gradually formed.

Among the notable centers of learning in the Russian Empire, which historically marked the beginning of national medical education, as well as the formation of the first collections of anatomical specimens, were Imperial Moscow University (IMU, opened in 1755), Imperial Kazan University (IKU, opened in 1804), and the Imperial Medical-Surgical Academy (IMSA, officially established on the order of Paul I in 1798).

The acquisition methods of IMSA relied on the financial support of the government, the royal family, and aristocratic benefactors. For example, in 1799 the Russian government set aside an annual amount of 5,000 rubles for the purpose of enlarging the anatomical collections of IMSA. Of great importance were donations by the royal family, and the Russian aristocracy, used to purchase collections from abroad. In 1820, Emperor Alexander I purchased a collection of wax pathological preparations from the Josephine Academy of Medicine at Vienna.[2] According to a directive of the Medical Collegium (the former Medical Chancellery), which was entrusted with the advancement of medical education, the IMHA received the following collections: the Johann Nathanael Liebekühn collection, which consisted of dry, alcoholic, and microscopic preparations; a collection of anatomical preparations from Count Zavadovsky; a selection of injectable preperations from the collection of F. Ruysch, which were not included in the Kunstkammer collection of the Russian Academy of Sciences; and a significant collection of human specimens demonstrating anatomical abnormalities, which was collected by the Medical Chancellery throughout the eighteenth century.[3] Unfortunately, many of the preparations from the collections mentioned above had to be excluded from the museum collections at the time of acquisition due to damage or deterioration.

A new development in the acquisition process for anatomical museums was the appearance of items that had a particular historical value. In the first half of the nineteenth century, historical items and even entire collections began to be secured with the intention of making Russian museums' holdings comprehensive. For example, IMSA purchased Professor Knackstedt's osteological collection in the 1800s, which, according to the Professor's will, was intended to be used in students' training in its entirety, rather than selectively. A new impetus to the development of the anatomical collections in IMSA was provided by Nikolai Ivanovich Pirogov (1810–1881), who became professor at the Academy in 1841. He created a new auxiliary education unit and expanded classrooms and museum-cabinets, demanding that the administration gather together all the preparations and bones, which had been scattered in different places, in order to create an integrated systematic collection, and provide three rooms for the museum. Anatomist V. L. Gruber (1814–1890), an assistant who later became Pirogov's successor, demonstrated unequaled skill in the art of anatomical preparations. Only some fragments of the anatomical preparations made by Gruber have been preserved in Russia up to the present day. His intense organizational activities at the Academy were marked by the construction of a new anatomical-physiological building in which special rooms were assigned for collections. Soon, however, the number of preparations significantly exceeded the space available to house them. Great credit goes to Professor of Normal Anatomy A. I. Tarenetskii (1845–1905) for the conservation, development, and restructuring of the anatomical collections of the IMSA. In accordance with anatomical views and the prevailing system of teaching anatomy at that time, the entire collection was divided into ten parts: bones and ligaments (1,920 items); ligaments, joints, and *bursae mucosae* and preparations showing the development of bones (100 items); the muscular collection (311 items); digestive organs (620 items); the respiratory system (162 items); the genitourinary system (300 items); the vascular system (645 items); the nervous system (123 items); the sensory system (263 items); and embryology and teratology (325 items).[4]

In the 1820s, the anatomical cabinet of Prof. J. C. Loder, a personal physician to Alexander I, was transported entirely to Russia and transferred to IMU by order of the Tsar. Such collections were carefully preserved as evidence of new developments in medical science and practice, as well as for supporting the ongoing research of foreign specialists who had relocated to Russia. These collections were stored in special cabinets, rooms, and halls of academic departments. Professors and teachers served as custodians of these collections, also allowing students to examine specimens for instructional purposes. Furthermore, under Loder's leadership, the holdings of the IMU anatomical museum reached 5,000 items in 1826.[5] He not only produced the preparations, but also acquired them from well-known European anatomists; these acquisitions included microscopic preparations. All the preparations were provided with specific numbers and very detailed descriptions. Unfortunately, only a few samples of the collection are extant. Also during this period the head of the IMU therapeutic clinic A.I. Over (1804–1864), a famous Moscow practitioner and a man of great talent, was conducting medical research of his own. In 1846, Over decided to unveil the wealth of material he had been collecting for over seventeen years and published his atlas of anatomical pathology *Selecta praxis medico-chirurgicale quam Mosquae exercet Alexander Auver* in Latin.[6] The atlas, with illustrations by the artist Shchyogolev, was well-received by the international community.[7] Over's collection has been partially preserved to the present day.

Outside of Moscow, a milestone for the academic medical community at IKU was the formation of the new Anatomical Theatre and University Clinic in the late 1830s–early 1840s, where their collections were permanently relocated for long-term preservation. In the second half of the nineteenth century, the osteological collections at IKU were expanded by undertaking complex archeological expeditions in the surrounding areas. The findings discovered during these expeditions later supplemented the core collection. In 1877 Sergei Mikhailovich Chugunov, a student of the medical faculty of IKU, discovered an old cemetery at the Simbirsk excavation site, called the "Old Crown."[8] He transported archeological findings from this site to the city of Kazan, where, under the guidance of Professor of Anatomy D.S. Yermolayev and anatomist N.M. Maliev (1841–1916), he made a detailed study of the craniums and took anthropological measurements of the remains that later became part of the IKU museum collections.

Beginning in the 1860s a number of exhibitions took place which were of great importance for the dissemination of medical knowledge in Russian society. Representatives of scientific societies and university professors served as the driving force behind their organization. The range of these medical exhibitions, consisting of scientific, industrial, and regional variants, was broad, covering the entire central part of the country. Contemporaries valued the importance of such medical collections very highly. For example, after visiting the Scientific and Industrial Exhibition in Kazan in 1890, S. Dyachenko, the Mayor of Kazan, raved, "These splendid collections were of great scientific interest and triggered the curiosity even of the least educated visitors. Although these exhibits, for the most part, were not simple enough for the understanding of lay people, they were important, however, as they popularized medical information at large and showed the considerable success that has been recently achieved in science."[9]

Anatomical collections played a role in both preparing for war and communicating its detrimental effects to the broader public. Regiments, reserve and regular battalions, military hospitals, and health facilities in European and Asiatic Russia received skeletons linked by maceration and hinges from IMSA for many years. Similar samples of skeletons and other preparations were made for a variety of educational and medical institutions in Russia and were exported abroad.[10] In 1896 the Russian branch of the Red Cross organized an anatomical exhibition that displayed a collection of skulls (65 items), damaged by small 8 mm caliber bullets, and bones (175 items), damaged by bullets common for that time, at their Pavilion in Nizhny Novgorod. This collection was compiled by Dr. K. Reier, who had served in several wars, and Professor E. V. Pavlov (1845–1916). In addition to war-damaged bones, shell-splinters and bullets extracted from the bodies of the soldiers and officers during surgical interventions were also exhibited. In broad terms, the exposition convincingly demonstrated to the public the destructive power of small arms on human bodies and undoubtedly spurred visitors to think not only about the horrible effects of the wounds, but also about the necessity of preventing military conflicts in the world. Thus, the exhibits of the medical department contributed greatly to the dissemination of ideas of charity and good-neighborly relations among countries. In the sector of private collections there was a particular interest in gathering medical items in order to document events that the collector himself or his contemporaries took part in. Current events had become an object of study to be preserved for posterity.

At present specimens in the collections of universities and medical schools exist only for the purposes of studying normal and pathological anatomy or for developing new surgical approaches and interventions. The "habitat" of osteological collections is currently limited to special rooms which are inaccessible to the public. They are rarely displayed for public viewing, since they are considered to be extremely *specific* material. Scientific and technical progress has opened the possibility of creating anatomical models from synthetic materials which are widely used for educational purposes. Artificial models and mannequins gradually superseded original bone remains for demonstrations to students. Original preparations of famous anatomists and surgeons, which are partially preserved, have been relegated to the historical part of these collections. Information on the development of osteological collections and other anatomical collections in Russia can be recovered via indirect documents, such as memoirs, our predecessors' research, or publications in periodicals. Only some collections of the Imperial period of Russian history were cataloged or officially noted in registration books. Even these documents have not been preserved completely.

Students' and researchers' work with authentic remains is being replaced by 3D computer models using special programs as a new visualizing method. The development of the plastination technique in the late twentieth and early twenty-first centuries has opened up new opportunities to the curators of anatomical collections.[11] Plastinated examples can be found at the Morphological Center of the S.M. Kirov Military Medical Academy in St. Petersburg and are distributed all over Russia, whereas bone remains have been moved to museum storage. The cataloging and careful maintenance of extant anatomical specimens, as well as of other parts of collections, are not a matter of priority for museum staff, and there is no funding available for this kind of work. Anatomy professors' individual initiative and sense of personal responsibility to our descendants were the main motivations for the restoration of Pirogov's preserved reparations, which was carried out in 2009 and 2010 at the Morphological Center under the supervision of Professor N.F. Fomin. Several external factors have had a negative impact on numerous anatomical collections that are preserved in medical institutions in the Russian Federation. If these collections were the main subject matter for research in the nineteenth century and were sometimes transferred to new media (i.e., by means of drawing, engraving, and photography), today they are not transferred to other forms of media for preservation (such as microscopic preparations, descriptive texts, photo, and/or video); they are also not registered and are rarely made from cadavers. Decaying exhibits are being disposed of and made to disappear forever, without leaving a trace. The preservation of human remains from archaeological excavations in the anthropological and ethnological collections of the state museums of the country is faring no better. Among the historic anatomical collections at the Medical University of Tomsk, wax dummies made by the company "Tramont" have been preserved in good condition until the present day and are still useful for students' education, but this is an example of the exception proving the rule. Models of human organs from papier-mâché and sketches, which were made more than a century ago, have acquired the status of rare objects and are preserved in greater numbers than the original osteological collections of the past.

The Leiden Declaration on Human Anatomy/Anatomical Collections adopted at the International Conference on Cultures of Anatomical Collections, held at Leiden University February 15–18, 2012, promptly drew the attention of the world scientific community to the need for speedy solutions to improve the rapidly deteriorating conditions that many anatomical collections are currently relegated to. The experience of our colleagues from the Coordinating Body for Scientific University Collections of Humboldt University in Berlin, Germany, concerning medical topics can serve as a guide for beginners who wish to make catalogs of anatomical collections available on the Internet, which will facilitate the kind of exchange of different perspectives and information that is indispensible for modern scholars.

NOTES

1. In Russian this government entity is called "Aptekarsky Prikaz."
2. Korovin, I., *Kratkii istoricheskii ocherk kafedry patologicheskoi anatomii pri Imperatorskoi Voenno-meditsinskoi (byvshei Mediko-Khirurgicheskoi) Akademii*, St. Petersburg: Narodnaia Pol'za, 1898, 8.
3. Ibid., 6–7.
4. Burlykina, M.I., *Muzei vysshikh uchebnykh zavedenii dorevoliutsionnoi Rossii (1724–1917 gody)*, Syktyvkar: Syktyvkarskii gos. universitet, 2000, 176.
5. Sapin, M.R., "Professora-anatomy i anatomicheskii muzei v MMA im. I.M. Sechenova," *Meditsinskaia professura Rossiiskoi Imperii. Kratkoe soderzhanie i tezisy dokladov nauchnoi konferentsii 3 marta 2006 g*, Moscow, 2006, 183.
6. Skorokhodov, L.Ia., *Kratkii ocherk istorii russkoi meditsiny*, Leningrad: Izd-vo "Prakticheskaia meditsina," 1926, 100.

7. "Over, Aleksandr Ivanovich," *Biographiia.ru: Biographicheskaia entsiklopediia*, http://www.biografija.ru/show_bio.aspx?id=99238. Accessed January 9, 2020.

8. Gorbunov, N.A., "Raskopki S.M. Chugunova na ploshchadi Staryi Venets v Simbirske v 1878 g," *Materialy chetvertoi nauchnoi konferentsii, posviashchennoi uchenomu i kraevedu S.L. Sytinu*, Ul'ianovsk: Izdatel'stvo "Korporatsiia tekhnologii prodvizheniia," 2008, 240–244.

9. *Otchet Komiteta Kazanskoi nauchno-promyshlennoi vystavki 1890 goda, sostoiashchei pod pokrovitel'stvom Ego Imperatorskogo Vysochestva gosudaria naslednika tsesarevicha,* Kazan', 1891, 24.

10. Tarenetskii, A., *Kafedra i muzei normal'noi anatomii pri Imperatorskoi Voenno-Meditsinskoi (byvshei Mediko-Khirurgicheskoi) Akademii v Sankt-Peterburge za 100 let. Istoricheskii ocherk,* St. Petersburg, 1895, 273.

11. This is the same technique used to create the specimens on display in the popular Body Worlds exhibits, which originated in Germany and now tour museums and exhibition sites worldwide (from the editors).

WORKS CITED

Burlykina, M.I. *Muzei vysshikh uchebnykh zavedenii dorevoliutsionnoi Rossii (1724–1917 gody)*. Syktyvkar: Syktyvkarskii gos. universitet, 2000.

Gorbunov, N.A. "Raskopki S.M. Chugunova na ploshchadi Staryi Venets v Simbirske v 1878 g." *Materialy chetvertoi nauchnoi konferentsii, posviashchennoi uchenomu i kraevedu S.L. Sytinu*. Ul'ianovsk: Izdatel'stvo "Korporatsiia tekhnologii prodvizheniia," 2008.

Korovin, I. *Kratkii istoricheskii ocherk kafedry patologicheskoi anatomii pri Imperatorskoi Voenno-meditsinskoi (byvshei Mediko-Khirurgicheskoi) Akademii*. St. Petersburg: Narodnaia Pol'za, 1898.

Otchet Komiteta Kazanskoi nauchno-promyshlennoi vystavki 1890 goda, sostoiashchei pod pokrovitel'stvom Ego Imperatorskogo Vysochestva gosudaria naslednika tsesarevicha. Kazan', 1891.

"Over, Aleksandr Ivanovich." *Biographiia.ru: Biographicheskaia entsiklopediia*. http://www.biografija.ru/show_bio.aspx?id=99238. Accessed January 9, 2020.

Sapin, M.R. "Professora-anatomy i anatomicheskii muzei v MMA im. I.M. Sechenova." *Meditsinskaia professura Rossiiskoi Imperii. Kratkoe soderzhanie i tezisy dokladov nauchnoi konferentsii 3 marta 2006 g*. Moscow, 2006.

Skorokhodov, L.Ia. *Kratkii ocherk istorii russkoi meditsiny*. Leningrad: Izd-vo "Prakticheskaia meditsina," 1926.

Tarenetskii, A. *Kafedra i muzei normal'noi anatomii pri Imperatorskoi Voenno-Meditsinskoi (byvshei Mediko-Khirurgicheskoi) Akademii v Sankt-Peterburge za 100 let. Istoricheskii ocherk.* St. Petersburg, 1895.

Chapter Three

The Doctor as a Humanist

An International, Interdisciplinary, and Intergenerational Project at Sechenov University

Jonathan McFarland and Irina Markovina

INTRODUCTION

As the Russian physician-writer Anton Chekhov (1860–1904) famously wrote, "medicine is my lawful wife, and literature my mistress; when I get tired of one, I spend the night with the other."[1] Although seemingly flippant, Chekhov's quotation is, in fact, pertinent on two counts. First, it illustrates his customary wit in the interweaving of the sciences (in this case, medicine) and the arts in late nineteenth- and early twentieth-century Russia. Chekhov, primarily speaking about his own personal relationship between his two sides, medicine and literature, unknowingly predicts and mirrors both Canadian physician and founding professor of Johns Hopkins Hospital William Osler (1849–1919), who said, "Twin berries on one stem, grievous damage has been done to both regarding the Humanities and Science in any other light than complemental,"[2] and then later American physician Arthur Kleinman who wrote, "Physicians are poised at the interface between scientific and lay cultures."[3] This balance between the arts (humanities) and the sciences has always been critically important.

But things began to change, and during the middle of the twentieth century this long-standing symbiotic relationship became increasingly unbalanced. C. P. Snow (1905–1980), when delivering the Rede lecture at Cambridge University, emphasized the widening chasm between the intellectual culture of science and the humanities.[4] Nobody would ever doubt that the enormous advances in the scientific side of medicine have led to great benefits for patients worldwide, both in diagnosis and in treatment. Nevertheless, this has meant that the humanities have taken a peripheral position, sometimes being disparagingly referred to as the *soft skills*.

Chekhov studied medicine at the Emperor's Moscow University Faculty of Medicine (now I. M. Sechenov First Moscow State Medical University, also called Sechenov University) from 1879 to 1884, when he graduated. During this time, in addition to studying medicine, he published short stories to maintain his family and help pay for his medical studies. It is worth noting that Chekhov began a research project for his doctoral thesis which was never published. Moreover, the theme of his research is relevant as he attempted to investigate Russian folklore and the history of the everyday life of the Russian people from a doctor's perspective. Doctor Chekhov, as opposed to Anton Pavlovich, was interested in the historical interpretation of disease and death, as well as how symptoms were interpreted and how healthcare providers were viewed by the Russian people. We could perhaps even suggest that Chekhov is the natural forerunner of narrative-based medicine.[5] The work, however, was never completed.

Some years later, however, he did manage to finish and later publish a work with a sociological-humanitarian slant related to his medical training and work. He spent around three months crossing Russia and Siberia, already ill with the tuberculosis that would later kill him, to reach Sakhalin Island, which was a penal colony. He spent another three months dedicated to reporting on the social conditions of life on the island. Geoffrey Borny states, "Chekhov may not have been a revolutionary, but in both medicine and literature he attempted to bring about change and improvement in life. His scientific research into the physical and social conditions then prevailing in the penal colony on the island of Sakhalin was only a small part of Chekhov's active approach to alleviating social ills."[6] Simon Karlinsky adds how "his life was one continuous round of alleviating famine, fighting epidemics, building schools . . . and hundreds of other pursuits designed to help his fellow man and improve the general quality around him."[7] Furthermore, this all occurred in a life considerably shortened by his disease, for he died aged only forty-four. Therefore, we hold Chekhov as an archetype both for his deeds as literary writer, medical practitioner, and social reformer and also for the fact that he started his medical career at Sechenov University, and, in this connection, we explain how we have tried to bring the humanities back to the core of medical education both at Sechenov University, and on the international stage. We have Anton Chekhov to thank, for to move forward we always need to look backward, or as Kierkegaard said, "Life can only be understood backwards; but it must be lived forwards."[8]

There are many historical figures in Russian culture who contributed to the field of medical humanities. We wish to mention a few here in order to outline the context of our project. First, there were writers with no medical background, but who made an important contribution to the development of the humanistic foundation of Russian medicine.[9] Second were medical doctors who were fundamental in managing to humanize spheres of human activity that had become synonymous with *in*humanity, such as war, prison, death, and even penal colonies, as with Chekhov's journey to Sakhalin. This is important to give context to the main section of this chapter, which discusses this new trend of developing medical humanities in Russia into international, interdisciplinary, and intergenerational projects, since the *new* is deeply rooted in the *old* (or the past)—in the historical achievements of outstanding figures coming from the fields of arts and medicine. And so, when talking of an introduction or integration of the humanities into medicine, we should always use the prefix "re." William Osler illustrated this well when he said, "the old art cannot possibly be *replaced by*, but must be *absorbed* in, the new science" (emphasis ours).[10]

The Russian perspective on the humanistic approach to healthcare is linked to many Russian doctors who are perhaps little known outside of Russia. We provide a brief desciption of these important figures below.

Doctor Matvei Mudrov (1776–1831) developed innovative strategies that introduced the basics of personalized, patient-centered medicine in Russia. Along these lines, he initiated reforms in medical education in Russia. In the beginning of the nineteenth century, he introduced the concept of palliative care into Russian healthcare practice.

Doctor Fyodor Haas (1780–1853) is well-known for his reforms of the prison healthcare system. He was named "Saint Doctor" by his patients. A well-off man at the beginning of his career, he died in poverty after having spent all his money on helping the poor. It is worth mentioning that one of his activities was publishing books for prisoners as well as books for children. He was one of the founders of a publishing house where he published his own book for children.

Doctor Nikolai Pirogov (1810–1881) is famous for his reforms in war medicine. He was the founder of Russian field surgery and developed the Russian school of anaesthesia. He was the first to use plaster casts to treat wounded soldiers. It was also he who introduced nursing care for the wounded during wartime.

Doctor Vyacheslav Manassein (1841–1901) is known for publishing the weekly newspaper *Vrach* (*The Physician*) where he, as chief editor, discussed the professional ethics of a doctor. Doctor Manassein was also the chairman of the Literary Foundation.

Luka Voyno-Yasenetsky (1877–1961) was an outstanding surgeon, a researcher, and writer on purulent surgery. He was also a spiritual writer and bishop of the Russian Orthodox Church who received the Stalin prize for surgery when he was Archbishop of Simferopol and the Crimea.

THE DOCTOR AS A HUMANIST PROJECT: DEVELOPING THE PRESENT

The question to be asked is why the medical humanities and why now? As Sir John Temple noted at a lecture at Sechenov University in April 2016, "medicine is not country-specific but global."[11] Iona Heath states, "evidence-based medicine [EBM] tempts us to try and describe people in terms of data from biomedical science; these are not and will never be, enough."[12] The attempt to treat the disease, or the pathological change that the patient consults the medical clinician for, is, we believe, only one half of the equation. Heath continues by saying, "such evidence is essential but always insufficient for the care of patients,"[13] for health professionals need to attempt to solve the whole equation and care for the patient who has the illness; this task includes taking into account the subjective perception of how the disease has affected, is affecting, and will affect the person. Heath finishes by explaining that EBM "gives us an alphabet, but as clinicians, we remain unsure of the language."[14] We believe that the humanities combined with the sciences enable the alphabet to produce a language that the clinician and patient can then use to communicate in unison. The humanities are needed to unlock the door, to allow the doctor to help the afflicted person as best as possible. As Sir William Osler emphasized more than a century ago, "the good physician treats the disease; the great physician treats the patient who has the disease."[15]

As has been shown, Russian medicine has always had a powerful tradition of applying humanistic principles in providing healthcare and in medical education. During the second half of the twentieth century special subjects (both compulsory and elective ones) directly relating to this humanistic tradition, for example, Bioethics and Medical Ethics, were introduced into the medical curriculum. This emphasis has been carried over to the present, as in the Current State Professional Educational Standards, that explain the competences that medical students should acquire during their medical training, the following criteria are included:

Students should be:

> "capable of analyzing socially significant issues and processes as well as applying the methods of the humanities, and the natural and medical-biological sciences in a variety of professional activities in their clinical practice." (General cultural competences of a doctor)[16]

> "capable of implementing ethical and deontological principles of the profession when communicating with colleagues, nurses and other medical care providers as well as with the adult population, teenagers, and their parents." (Professional competences of a doctor)[17]

Within this context, The Doctor as a Humanist initiative was born, both within Russia, predominantly at Sechenov University, and outside of Russia. This project is an illustration of a completely new trend in the development of modern Russian medical education. Physician training is being transformed based on the idea of combining the Russian and international approaches to medical education, opening up to the global professional community and fostering collaboration with universities in all parts of the world. Now more than ever medicine has become international: international teams undertake combined research, knowledge is accumulated and disseminated internationally, diseases in different regions of the world are combatted via joint efforts of doctors from different countries—this is the twenty-first century. And this is the only way to move forward in medical education, practice, and research. That is why our project, which is based at Sechenov, a Russian medical university, is implemented in English by an international, interdisciplinary, and intergenerational team.

The Doctor as a Humanist is an international and multicultural initiative aiming to help *return the heart and soul to medicine*. Its main objective is to promote the humanities in medical education and practice, to bridge theory and practice. The Doctor as a Humanist promotes cultural values in medical practice by advancing dialogue between the humanities and the biomedical sciences; its forte is that it is international, interdisciplinary, and intergenerational. It has developed into a multifaceted and yet holistic project that includes components such as extracurricular university training, international symposia, master classes, workshops and presentations at international conferences, journal publications and themed issues of journals, webinars, and even Special Interest Groups (SIGs) within the Association for Medical Education in Europe (AMEE).

Our first step was to introduce a School of Excellence on Humanism called the "Doctor as a Humanist" for medical students at Sechenov University in 2017. Interestingly enough, there are a number of Schools of Excellence at Sechenov University, for example, in Internal Medicine, Innovation Methods in Anatomic Pathology, Surgical Obstetrics, Fetal Medicine, Medical Dentistry, Methodology of Diagnosis in Psychiatry, etc. The students choose a school that meets their special interests in the medical profession, apply, compete, and are enrolled to acquire in-depth knowledge and skills to become better doctors in the future. However, ours broke that mold and to some extent was revolutionary since it was the first time in the university that students were offered training in a non-clinical subject, and that the language of instruction was English.

The Doctor as a Humanist School of Excellence used a blended learning approach. The majority of the sessions were held online using Skype as the lecturer was based in Spain, but both the start and the finish of the course were held at Sechenov University at the Institute of Linguistics. We based the course on the textbook *Medical Humanities: An Introduction* by Nathan Carlin, Ronald A. Carson, and Thomas R. Cole and divided it into six sections: history and medicine, literature and medicine, cinema and medicine, studying medicine, philosophy and medicine, and religion and medicine. A great deal of emphasis was placed on allowing the students to present and discuss works of literature or topics we believed could be of interest to them. Indeed, many students commented that in the online sessions they could freely discuss many topics that during their day-to-day studies they had no opportunity to explore; something that should be commented on is the importance of making this course *relevant* to the students' studies. For instance, during the section devoted to history students worked in pairs on topics that arose from *The BMJ*'s issue on Medical Milestones. There were fascinating talks on such topics as evidence-based medicine, birth control pills, tissue culture, and so on. When we discussed literature, students wrote reflective essays on such works as *A Leg to Stand On* (Oliver Sacks), *Darkness Visible: A Memoir of Madness* (William Styron), and *The Diving Bell and the Butterfly* (Jean Dominique Bauby). We were very lucky in that for one session we had the physician and author Gavin Francis attend and discuss his book, *Adventures in Human Being: A Grand Tour From the Cranium to the Calceneum*. At the end of course students gave oral presentations on a range of subjects such as "Aging in Films," "Famous Writers in Medicine," "Buddhism and Medicine," and even "The Importance of Rene Guenon." However, the course, and indeed The Doctor as a Humanist project as a whole, is for the students, and their opinions are always interesting and important to take into account, and this case is no exception:

> I would like to take part in the school "The Doctor as a Humanist" because it is a golden opportunity to receive new knowledge in philosophy, ethics, history and literature. In my opinion, these branches of science are necessary for every modern doctor. (4th year student)

> Nowadays there is a very delicate balance between the "scientific" and the "humanistic." It is very easy to get carried away with new ideas and forget about basic humanistic truths in the twenty-first century, in the century of rapidly advancing technologies. There is a struggle in every doctor, and everyone decides what kind of doctor he or she wants to be. . . . I believe that humanism is a partially innate quality and at the same time an essential part of a well-bred person. But even if this is so, we can and should cultivate humanism in ourselves and constantly set our minds on self-improvement. (4th year student)

> In my opinion, reading literature may be considered a kind of conversation, too. Writers have the advantage of expressing their experience, thoughts, mistakes and advice with considerable elegance, as well as humor and irony which can make any conversation memorable and pleasant. Reading Mikhail Bulgakov's *A Country Doctors' Notebook*, for example, was as satisfying and useful as talking to a peer about his or her both successful and awkward interactions. Reading helps one to reconsider his or her own priorities, as well as to gain a fresh look at moral problems that may have insidiously haunted me. (6th year student)

As part of the project, the first International Symposium "The Doctor as a Humanist" was held (October 13–14, 2017) in Palma de Mallorca and was excellently received. Many illustrious speakers from Europe, North America, and Asia participated, all united by a common bond to develop a more humanistic medicine. The Symposium was opened with the subtitle "Can the humanities transform the medicine of the twenty-first century?" The success of the Symposium was the result of cooperation between lecturers from five European and American universities: Sechenov University (Moscow), Pompeu Fabra University (Barcelona), Queens University (Belfast), the University of the Balearic Islands (Palma), and Johns Hopkins University (Baltimore), and experts in medical humanities and education from the United Kingdom, Spain, Russia, Brazil, India, the United States, and Canada. It was organized by the Scientific Foundation of the Medical Council of the Balearic Islands in the Royal Academy of Medicine of the Balearic Islands.

It is critical to highlight that The Doctor as a Humanist does not purport to be a hierarchical project but one that is based on the ideas, initiatives, and tireless enthusiasm of the younger generation: the students and young doctors and professionals. With this in mind, their input has always been fundamental to the way of thinking of The Doctor as a Humanist, so at the first Symposium medical students participated by giving talks to a range of international experts. And this initial Symposium led to the first The Doctor as a Humanist Online Course (February to April 2019), a series of interactive webinars combining lectures, discussions, and student presentations prepared as home assignments that dealt with, among other topics: New Technologies and Dehumanization, Emotional Intelligence, Lyricism and Criticism in Opera, as well as Narrative Medicine, Mindfulness in Medicine, and Classical Indian Dance in Psychiatry. These webinars served as a place of exhibition and debate on highly topical issues, which require a more human vision from the doctor. In addition to an array of international speakers, students from Sechenov and Krasnoyarsk in Russia, as well as from various universities in Spain, Italy, Mexico, and Pakistan, among others, participated.

The Second International Symposium "The Doctor as a Humanist" (April 1–3, 2019) was held in Moscow at Sechenov University, the oldest and most prestigious Russian medical school, with more than 260 years of history. Once again researchers, professors, and doctors participated (and of course medical students this time, too) from three prestigious Spanish universities: the Pompeu Fabra University, the Autonomous University of Madrid, and the University of Les Iles Balears. In this new 2019 edition participation was higher than in 2017. At the second Symposium medical students, nursing professionals, and medical professors from the following institutions also participated: Oxford University and University of Glasgow (United Kingdom); Aalborg University (Denmark); Hamburg University (Germany); Johns Hopkins University (United States); and McGill University (Canada), among others.

This second Symposium was even more international and ambitious than that of 2017, with the scientific program including roundtable discussions and presentations related to the incorporation of literature, painting, philosophy, music, and even dance in medical education. The active participation of medical students from diverse medical schools, led by the students from Sechenov University, was paramount to the success of the event. In addition to doctors and surgeons, a large group of nurses, professors, and deans of medical schools, as well as experts from publications such as *The BMJ*, joined the Symposium. And as we believe that you should practice what you preach, in addition to the talks, discussion panels, and posters, there was also time for social events with chamber music, guided tours at museums (e.g., the Bulgakov Museum), and other cultural activities, such as attending the opera *Don Pasquale* at the Bolshoi Theater. One of the long-term objectives of this initiative, which is integrated into the project's broader pedagogical purpose, is to create an International Association of Humanities and Medicine. Among other things, it should facilitate innovative ways to reintroduce more of the humanities into medical school curricula and clinical practice, as well as support collaboration between medical schools and encourage multidisciplinary and multisectoral cooperation. As a final goal, The Doctor as a Humanist aims to improve the practice of medicine by promoting the humanities in healthcare, and to restore the balance between the sciences and the humanities for, as we have seen, this balance existed in the past. The project is becoming more global and the Third International Symposium took place at Anáhuac University in Mexico City, Mexico (March 25–28, 2020). The central issue continues to be the transformative capacity of humanistic training in the practice of medicine, seeking greater consolidation of this movement through building bridges between cultures, disciplines, and generations.

CONCLUSION

"Potentially, the medical humanities do not simply add value to medical education by shifting an instrumental training into a values-oriented education, but, incorporated into the curriculum as core and integrated study, they can represent a critical rejoinder to a potentially reductive biomedicine that treats isolated symptoms rather than the person in context."[18] The authors believe that Bleakeley's words are more relevant now than ever before; the humanities are needed to restore balance to a medical curriculum (and thus practice) currently biased in favor of the sciences but the humanities cannot be seen as an added-on subject; they must be fully integrated. For, as Williams et al. comment, "A significant criticism of medical education over recent decades is that we focus on the disease"; and as they rightly continue, "The most fundamental of the arguments in favor of medical humanities, is that they may allow or validate a greater understanding of the human condition as part of medicine."[19] Medicine is practiced by people for people,[20] not yet by AI or robots, and the medical humanities can contribute to so much that is at stake in medical education, such as critical thinking, the importance of empathy and diversity, a global vision of health, disease, and illness, professionalism, communication abilities, and many more.

In a recent article Morera Serna writes, "Humanistic education helps to cope with the ups and downs of daily clinical work building resilient physicians. Investing in Medical Humanities to achieve top professionals may be one of the soundest ideas of medical schools."[21] We appreciate and wholeheartedly agree with the sentiment of this practicing physician. Twenty-first-century medicine is not confined to individual countries but is a global concern, and Russia is now opening up to the world stage in medical education, with the project mentioned in this chapter, The Doctor as a Humanist, being a very good example, with its principal aim of helping medical students and young doctors become incorporated in the international professional community. And perhaps, the best strategy—as we see it—would be to remember the achievements of the *past*, analyze the state of things in the *present*, and based on that, be prepared for the *future*. Now is most definitely the time to "ensure that the Medical Humanities do not remain" "a castle in the air."[22] As we have noted previously, "The stakes are too high. The future of medicine depends on finding the way to (re)introduce the humanities to the core of medical education."[23] And, for the authors, The Doctor as a Humanist has started to take the small steps needed to achieve this goal.

NOTES

1. The Russian versions of Chekhov's letters are from the Academy edition of Chekhov's *Polnoe sobranie pisem v 12 tomakh*, Moscow: Khudozhestvennaia literatura, 1974–83. This quotation is from a letter to Alexei Suvorin, Volume II, 326.

2. Osler, William, "The Old Humanities and the New Science: The Presidential Address Delivered Before the Classical Association at Oxford, May 1919," *Br Med J* 1919, Jul 5;2 (3053): 1–7, 4.

3. Kleinman, Arthur, *The Illness Narratives: Suffering, Healing and the Human Condition*, New York: Basic Books, 1988, 241.

4. Snow, C.P., *The Two Cultures and the Scientific Revolution,* New York: Cambridge University Press, 1998.

5. For more on this topic, see Miller's chapter in the present volume.

6. Borny, Geoffrey, *Interpreting Chekhov*, Canberra: ANU Press, 2006, 25.

7. Chekhov, A.P., S. Karlinsky, and M.H. Heim, *Letters of Anton Chekhov*, New York: Harper & Row, 1973, 26.

8. Kierkegaard, *Journals* IV A 164, 1843.

9. Works by Fyodor Dostoyevsky (1821–1881), Leo Tolstoy (1828–1910), and later by Anton Chekhov and Mikhail Bulgakov—to mention just a few—changed Russian society, as well as created the ideological (in the best sense of the word) context for the development of humanistic tradition in the Russian medical care and education.

10. Osler, William, "The Reserves of Life," *St Mary's Hospital Gazette* (1907) 13: 95–98.

11. Temple, Sir John. Lecture given at Sechenov University, April 2016.

12. Heath, Iona, "How Medicine Has Exploited Rationality at the Expense of Humanity: An Essay by Iona Heath," *The BMJ* (2016): 355.

13. Heath, "How Medicine Has Exploited Rationality at the Expense of Humanity: An Essay by Iona Heath," 355.

14. Heath, "How Medicine Has Exploited Rationality at the Expense of Humanity: An Essay by Iona Heath," 355.

15. Cited in Shorter, Edward, "Primary Care," *The Cambridge Illustrated History of Medicine*, Ed. Roy Porter, Cambridge, Cambridge University Press, 2001, 118–153, 144.

16. A copy of these state guidelines in Russian may be found at the following link: https://www.s-vfu.ru/universitet/rukovodstvo-i-struktura/instituty/mi/u/oop/RPD%20Pf/%D0%A0%D0%9F%D0%94_%D0%A1%D1%82%D0%BE%D0%BC%D0%B0%D1%82%D0%BE%D0%BB%D0%BE%D0%B3%D0%B8%D1%8F_%D0%9F%D0%A4.pdf, p. 3–4.

17. A copy of these state guidelines in Russian may be found at the following link: http://chelsma.ru/files/misc/pk-1ped.pdf, p. 3.

18. Bleakeley, A., "When I Say . . . The Medical Humanities in Medical Education," *Medical Education* (2015) 49.6: 959–960.

19. Williams, Eleri and A. Neil Turner, "Broadening Our Horizons: Are Medical Humanities an Essential Part of Medical Education?," *Nephrology Dialysis Transplantation* (2018) 33.9: 1511–1513, 1511.

20. Liao, L., "Opening Our Eyes to a Critical Approach to Medicine: The Humanities in Medical Education," *Medical Teacher* (2017) 39.2: 220–221, 220.

21. Morera Serna, Eduardo, "Medical Humanities in a Rapidly Changing World. Is There Any Worth in It?," *MedEdPublish* (2018) 7 [3], 54.

22. Wu, H. and J. Chen, "Conundrum Between Internationalisation and Interdisciplinarity: Reflection on the Development of Medical Humanities in Hong Kong, Taiwan and China," *MedEdPublish* (2018) 7 [3], 46.

23. McFarland, J., I. Markovina, and T. Gibbs, "Concluding Commentary. The Importance of the Humanities in Medical Education: Where Are We Now?," *MedEdPublish* (2018) 7 [3], 83.

WORKS CITED

Bleakeley, A. "When I Say . . . The Medical Humanities in Medical Education," *Medical Education* (2015) 49.6: 959–960.

Borny, Geoffrey. *Interpreting Chekhov*. Canberra: ANU Press, 2006.

Chekhov, A.P., S. Karlinsky, and M.H. Heim. *Letters of Anton Chekhov*. New York: Harper & Row, 1973.

Chekhov, A.P. *Polnoe sobranie pisem v 12 tomakh*. Moscow: Khudozhestvennaia literatura, 1974–83.

Heath, Iona. "How Medicine Has Exploited Rationality at the Expense of Humanity: An Essay by Iona Heath," *The BMJ* (2016): 355.

Kierkegaard, Soren. *Journals* IV A 164, 1843.

Kleinman, Arthur. *The Illness Narratives: Suffering, Healing and the Human Condition*, New York: Basic Books, 1988.

Liao, L. "Opening Our Eyes to a Critical Approach to Medicine: The Humanities in Medical Education," *Medical Teacher* (2017) 39.2: 220–221.

McFarland, J., I. Markovina, and T. Gibbs, "Concluding Commentary. The Importance of the Humanities in Medical Education: Where Are We Now?," *MedEdPublish* (2018) 7 [3], 83.

Morera Serna, Eduardo. "Medical Humanities in a Rapidly Changing World. Is There Any Worth in It?," *MedEdPublish* (2018) 7 [3], 54.

Osler, William. "The Old Humanities and the New Science: The Presidential Address Delivered Before the Classical Association at Oxford, May 1919." *Br Med J* 1919, Jul 5; 2 (3053): 1–7.

Osler, William. "The Reserves of Life." *St Mary's Hospital Gazette* (1907) 13: 95–98.

Shorter, Edward. "Primary Care." *The Cambridge Illustrated History of Medicine*. Ed. Roy Porter. Cambridge, Cambridge University Press, 2001. 118–153.

Snow, C.P. *The Two Cultures and the Scientific Revolution.* New York: Cambridge University Press, 1998.

Temple, Sir John. Lecture given at Sechenov University, April 2016.

Williams, Eleri and A. Neil Turner, "Broadening Our Horizons: Are Medical Humanities an Essential Part of Medical Education?," *Nephrology Dialysis Transplantation* (2018) 33.9: 1511–1513.

Wu, H. and J. Chen, "Conundrum Between Internationalisation and Interdisciplinarity: Reflection on the Development of Medical Humanities in Hong Kong, Taiwan and China," *MedEdPublish* (2018) 7 [3], 46.

Chapter Four

Chekhov in North American Medical Schools

Surveying the Pre-COVID Attitudes of Slavic Scholars and Their Role in Medical Humanities

Konstantin Starikov

BACKGROUND

In the last sixty years the field of medical humanities has become firmly established as a valued and pragmatic application of interdisciplinary studies from the liberal arts in a variety of academic and non-academic settings, including hospitals and clinical practices. Closely related to the missions of bioethics and moral education, medical humanities (or health humanities as a broader discipline) are faced with the challenge of raising difficult questions about the human condition. Martin Kohn, Associate Professor of Medicine and Director of the Program in Medical Humanities in the Center for Ethics, Humanities and Spiritual Care at the Cleveland Clinic, explains the difference between bioethicists and medical humanists in terms of humanists' tolerance for uncertainty and ambiguity: "They (bioethicists) seek to resolve patient and provider value-driven problems; we (medical humanists), in turn, ask problematic questions about the human condition that have no definite answers."[1]

It is this tolerance for ambiguity that programs in medical humanities attempt to introduce into a biomedical worldview from the vantage point of the empathetic doctor. Rita Charon (MD, PhD in English literature), a pioneer in narrative medicine, considers ambiguity as "a constant in our work and a required aspect of our teaching and practice of close reading."[2]

Verbal communication plays a central role in medical encounters, and, in order to act meaningfully, the value of tolerance for ambiguity needs to be systematically explored in medical education with the aim of preparing future doctors to strengthen the doctor-patient relationship. It is in this context that Anton Chekhov's observation about the art of writing reveals his training as a physician, as the medical profession especially relies on the stories of illness. In a letter to his editor Chekhov wrote: "You are right in demanding that an artist should take an intelligent attitude to his work, but you confuse two things: solving a problem and stating a problem correctly. It is only the second that is obligatory for the artist. In *Anna Karenina* and *Evgeny Onegin* not a single problem is solved, but they satisfy you completely because all the problems are correctly stated in them. It is the business of the judge to put the right questions, but the answers must be given by the jury according to their own preference." (Anton Chekhov to Alexei Suvorin, October 27, 1888).[3]

One of my early observations about the field of medical humanities was the frequent inclusion of short stories by Chekhov (1860–1904) and Lev Tolstoy (1828–1910) in courses, seminars, and workshops, which are usually conducted by medical practitioners.[4]

According to my review of course syllabi and workshop programs available online, Tolstoy's story *The Death of Ivan Ilych* is perhaps one of the most widely used literary texts in discussions of death on medical campuses and in hospitals. Although not as predominant as Tolstoy's story, Chekhov's short stories are used by instructors to spark discussions about poverty, social injustice, public health, and the doctor-patient relationship. Commentaries on Russian writers, including the famous doctor-writers such as Chekhov and Mikhail Bulgakov (1891–1940), are published in peer-reviewed medical and public health journals.

Medical humanists reflect on the engagement of medicine and the humanities in terms of bridging the gap between "the two cultures," as C. P. Snow (1905–1980) characterized science and the humanities in his influential lecture, subsequently published as *The Two Cultures and the Scientific Revolution*. In the 1960s and 1970s physicians and humanists started a reform movement that attempted to remedy the threat (at least this is how it was perceived by educators and bioethicists) of the dehumanization of medicine. Since then the shared view has been that the ideal of the doctor who was well-read in Greek and Latin no longer reflected the spirit of modern medicine and that an undergraduate liberal arts education was not effective preparation for solving the problems of the commercialization of medicine. As a result, the following excerpt from Edmund Pellegrino's essay "Medical Humanism and Technological Anxiety," based on the lecture he delivered in Michigan in 1976, retains its relevancy today, in the first half of the twenty-first century:

> Medical humanism has achieved the status of a salvation theme, which can absolve the perceived sins of modern medicine. The catalogue of those "sins" is long, varied, and often contradictory: overspecialization; technicism; overprofessionalization; insensitivity to personal and socio-cultural values; too narrow a construal of the doctor's role; too much "curing" rather than "caring"; not

> enough emphasis on prevention, patient participation, and patient education; too much science; too much economic incentive; a "trade school" mentality; insensitivity to the poor and socially disadvantaged; overmedicalization of everyday life; inhumane treatment of medical students; overwork by house staff; deficiencies in verbal and non-verbal communication. No list can be complete. Every conceivable failing is admissible in the critique of so human-centered an endeavor as medicine.[5]

An influential advocate of medical humanities, Edmund Pellegrino (1920–2013) made a point similar to Chekhov's emphasis on the spiritual mission of an author. Pellegrino emphasized the co-existence of medicine and literature in the preface to *Medicine and Literature*, edited by Enid Rhodes Peschel: "Medicine and literature are united in unremitting paradox; the need simultaneously to stand back from, and yet to share in, the struggle for human life. . . . Both of them are moral experiences. . . . To look compassionately is the summit of artistry for both medicine and literature; to take part in the struggle is the morality they share."[6]

Chekhov's medical education, too, allowed him to unite medicine and literature in a unique stylistic blend of poetic worldview and a critique of social ills in the tradition of Russian realism. In his autobiographical note, Chekhov wrote: "There is no doubt in my mind that my study of medicine has had a serious impact on my literary activities. It significantly broadened the scope of my observations and enriched me with knowledge whose value for me as a writer only a doctor can appreciate. It also served as a guiding influence; my intimacy with medicine probably helped me to avoid many mistakes. My familiarity with the natural sciences and scientific methods has always kept me on my guard; I have tried whenever possible to take scientific data into account, and where it has not been possible I have preferred not writing at all."[7]

If there is a consensus among medical humanists that Chekhov's short stories are useful to teach empathy to medical students, is there then a common point of view among Slavic scholars, especially those specializing in the nineteenth century and Chekhov in particular, on their own teaching practices in the non-medical setting? Is there an awareness of the challenges of teaching Chekhov to medical students? Do Slavic scholars think that they have a role in the rapidly growing field of medical humanities? Should Slavic departments develop special courses for the undergraduates interested in premedical concentrations?

My purpose in writing this chapter is to stimulate Slavic scholars to discuss these questions. The decline in the enrollment in Slavic language and literature courses over the past two decades has been attributed to the end of the Cold War and, at times, has also been blamed on trends in the gradual decline in enrollments across the humanities in general. The field of medical humanities offers a unique opportunity for Slavic scholars to develop a novel approach to the teaching of Chekhov in North American educational institutions. Some of the courses currently taught by faculty in the field of Slavic Studies would fit well in the advancement of skills required of future doctors. Other courses, not necessarily taught around medical themes, offer meaningful insights into the personal stories of illness and a philosophical analysis of medical issues from the point of view of narrative ethics, and, therefore, may be offered as electives to a wider audience of medical students.

The interdisciplinary nature of medical humanities, in my view, would allow Slavic scholars to collaborate not only with doctors but also with digital humanists. The prevalence of new technologies in medicine, including data visualizations, offers exploration with tools that enrich close readings with distant readings. Exploring reading experiences with fMRI and PET technologies, such as the cognitive regulation of emotion when reading Chekhov, can add valuable insight into the teaching of empathy in the classroom. Collaborative partnerships with medical humanities programs may also open new venues for the teaching of Russian classics in a non-traditional setting. Because human experience is expressed through the narrative mode, Slavic scholars trained in the analysis of subjective narrative stories can make a lasting contribution to the contextualized teaching of doctor-writers like Chekhov.

METHOD

Before proposing a model of teaching Chekhov's short stories in medical education it is essential to understand current practices and attitudes of Slavic scholars specializing in the nineteenth and twentieth centuries, particularly in Chekhov studies, as well as to study their current awareness of medical humanities. With this purpose I created a questionnaire consisting of six questions among North American faculty mainly with a specialization in nineteenth century. The survey was conducted in 2017 via email correspondence, allowing me to eliminate questions about affiliation and faculty status. The email format was also meant to personalize the invitation to complete the survey and encourage responders to provide a more detailed explanation other than a "YES" or a "NO" response.

In total 30 respondents participated in the survey, comprising a hand-selected pool of faculty (a response rate of 50 percent). My sample selection was based on an environmental scan of faculty in the Slavic Literatures and Languages departments, conducted by searching staff directories of North American departmental websites and by identifying faculty whose scholarly interests included Chekhov or nineteenth-century Russian literature. I also conducted searches using the Google search engine using the following keywords: Chekhov, medical humanities, syllabus. The final sample group consisted of 60 individuals. Those Slavic faculty who are employed by institutions with an affiliated medical school were given priority for inclusion in the final sample. Answers were organized and tagged using Microsoft Excel. The respondents and references to respondents' institutions were also anonymized in order to protect privacy and obtain unbiased opinions.

SURVEY QUESTIONS

Q1: Do you have a medical humanities program at your institution?

Q2: Have you taught an undergraduate course in which you have incorporated Slavic literary texts relevant to the field of medical humanities?

Q3: Have you taught a graduate course or a workshop in which you have incorporated Slavic literary texts relevant to the study of medical humanities?

Q4: Have you taught a course or a workshop to the medical students or hospital staff in which you have incorporated Slavic literary texts relevant to the study of medical humanities?

Q5: If you were to include Chekhov's stories in your coursework (for any class) for teaching topics related to medical humanities, what are the top five?

Q6: Do you think Slavic literary scholars should have a role in medical education?

RESULTS

Q1

The summary of responses is shown below using a bar chart. Out of eight "YES" responses, one respondent explained that the program at his or her institution is "Health Humanities." The terms "Medical Humanities" and "Health Humanities" are often used interchangeably, however the proponents of the latter term argue that a broader umbrella term is more receptive to the inclusion of other medical professions such as dentists, nurses, psychologists, public health practitioners, and other professionals in healthcare. For our purposes, we treated the answer "Health Humanities" as an affirmative answer.

It is telling that all eight respondents are aware of the medical humanities programs as official programs. The academic institutions which employ these Slavic faculty have medical schools.

Out of thirteen "NO" answers seven respondents included qualifying comments which demonstrated an additional level of awareness about medical humanities at his or her institution. For example, one respondent indicated that a course on Medical Spanish is offered, which in his/her mind was relevant to the teaching of medical humanities but did not mention or did not know that this course was offered by the Department of Medical Humanities and Social Sciences. I was unable to verify by visiting a website the existence of an official program in medical humanities at that particular institution. Another respondent whose institution was planning to offer a Medical Humanities seminar (2017–2018) gave the answer "No, not yet," which implies that in the respondent's mind there is a possibility or perhaps even a prediction that such a program might be offered in the near future. The awareness of the discussions about the benefits of such a program is demonstrated by two other respondents: "No, not yet, but the university is considering launching one," and, "No, [my institution] does not have a medical humanities program at present." Two other answers implied uncertainty, which perhaps is framed by the existence of medical schools: "No, not to my knowledge" and "No, as far as I know." Because the structure of this question was designed to obtain a short positive or a negative answer rather than a detailed response one should not overgeneralize when interpreting these comments.

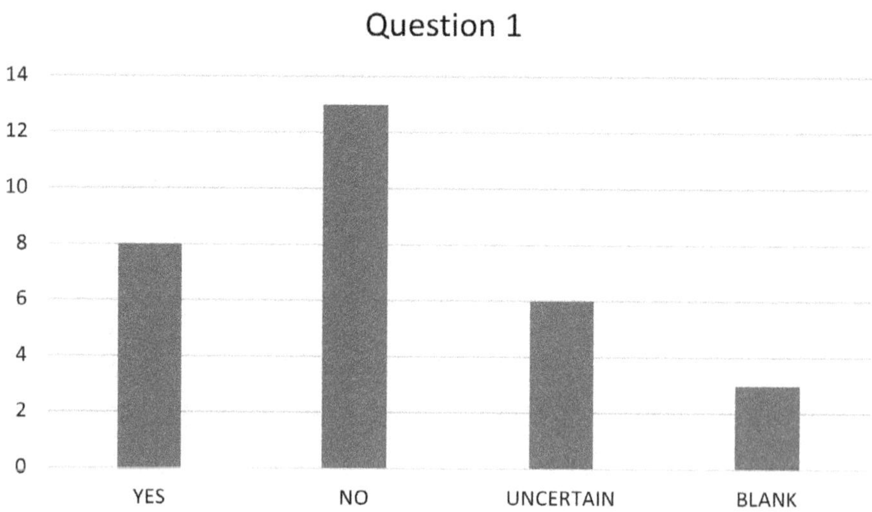

Figure 4.1. Question 1 Responses
Source: Konstantin Starikov

Six responses are categorized as "UNCERTAIN" because a respondent did not say "YES" or "NO." The qualitative comments clarify somewhat a respondent's awareness of the presence (or lack of) of a program in medical humanities. One respondent explained that there was a seminar on the topic at the Center for Humanities but because it was a few years ago and it was not offered regularly he or she is not aware of the program in medical humanities. A similar answer was given using the phrase "Not that I know of" which leans toward the answer "NO," including the answer "Not that I know of but I am not 100 percent sure." Two respondents said that they did not know. Three respondents did not provide an answer.

Q2

Out of a total of seventeen "YES" answers ten respondents provided an affirmative answer without any comments. Seven respondents supplemented their response with additional information about their teaching experience. One respondent indicated that s/he taught an undergraduate Literature and Medicine course. Other respondents described courses they have taught related to medical humanities: Madness and Power in Russia; Medical Ethics and End of Life Care. The reading lists included works by Nikolai Gogol (1809–1852), Ivan Turgenev (1818–1883), Tolstoy and Bulgakov.

Besides Chekhov, the frequency of using Tolstoy's and Bulgakov's literary texts in coursework is one of the highest. The respondents did not specify which texts were assigned for reading except Tolstoy's *Death of Ivan Ilych*, which a respondent said was useful "in training for medical practitioners working in hospice care." Another respondent explained that s/he used Tolstoy's texts dealing with death and illness. The topic of death and illness is not necessarily treated as a medical humanities topic, though. One respondent qualified the answer with the following observation: "Yes, although I did not make this relevance explicit when teaching these texts (examples include Gogol, Turgenev, Bulgakov, and, of course, Chekhov)." A more detailed analysis is required based on the survey of syllabi in order to gauge the prevalence of medical humanities as a conceptual category in courses offered in Slavic departments. Judging from the following comment the medical themes are used not only in literature courses but also in language teaching courses: "Yes, I do teach some very basic medical topics in Russian language courses. In my culture course we address issues of public health in Russia. In my literature classes we discussed mental health, spiritual health, and, when we cover Chekhov's work, the practice of medicine in nineteenth century Russia."

Out of ten "NO" answers, two respondents left explanations that might help us understand the fine distinction in perception of the offered course as relevant to medical humanities but not, at least in the instructor's mind,

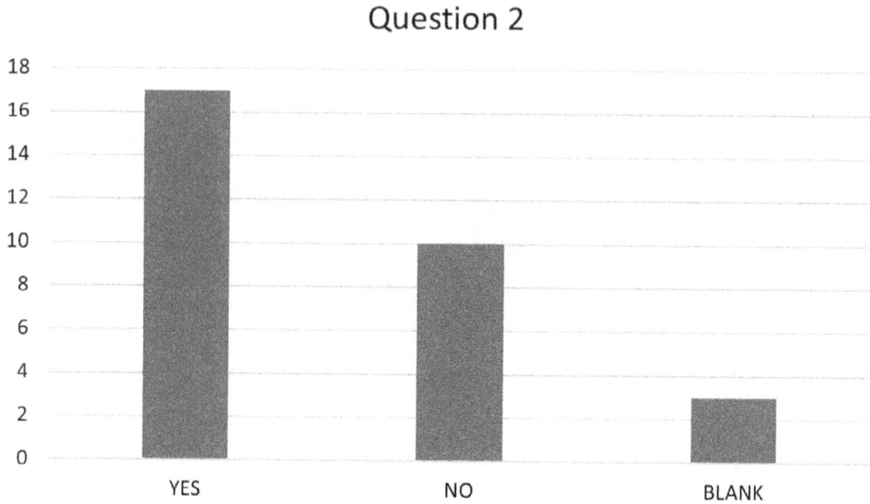

Figure 4.2. Question 2 Responses
Source: Konstantin Starikov

categorized as a course designed for a medical humanities program. For example, one respondent said that s/he assigns "some critical sources on Chekhov's 'debt to medicine,' but nothing to constitute a medical humanities approach." This comment raises a question about whether or not Slavic scholars who are interested in teaching in the field of medical humanities would want additional training in order to feel comfortable in approaching a medical humanities program with a class proposal. Similarly, an awareness that there is a growing interest in medical humanities might also help Slavic scholars to design courses with pre-medical students and those students interested in the biomedical sciences in purview. One respondent wrote, "I have attended more closely to Chekhov's analysis of class when I have taught his stories than to his treatment of medicine proper, although I suppose this too is a proper topic of medical humanities."

Q3

Six respondents answered that they have taught a graduate course or a workshop in which they incorporated Slavic literary texts relevant to the study of medical humanities. The question did not ask to name these texts and none of the respondents specified which texts they used or if these were Chekhov's short stories. One course was offered to both undergraduate and graduate students. Another was an interactive workshop with a paper presentation on *The Tragic Menagerie* by Lydiia Zinov'eva-Annibal (1886–1907).

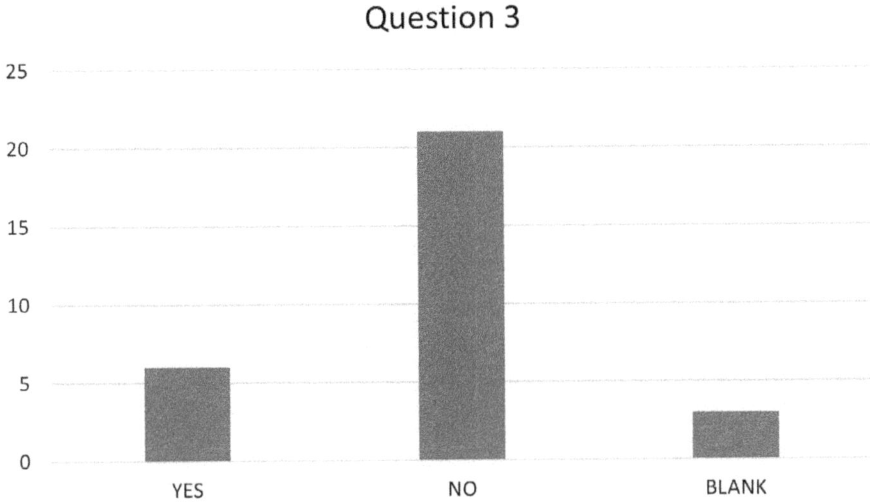

Figure 4.3. Question 3 Responses
Source: Konstantin Starikov

The majority of respondents answered "NO" to this question, which suggests that graduate students in Slavic departments are not exposed to the interdisciplinary field of medical humanities through their graduate coursework. It is also noteworthy that medical students who might be interested in taking a course involving a Slavic scholar are excluded from the offering of graduate courses in the humanities unless there is a special arrangement or an established medical humanities program with a liaison to a Slavic department. One respondent qualified his/her answer with a projection into the future, explaining that she will offer a medical humanities–related course at the graduate level. Another respondent who said that his/her institution does not have a graduate program in Slavic studies therefore implied that a medical humanities course by faculty in the Slavic department would be contingent on administrative support.

Q4

As expected, the total number of respondents who answered "YES" to the question regarding teaching a course or a workshop to medical students or hospital staff in which they incorporated Slavic literary texts relevant to the study of medical humanities was very low. Out of three responses, only one respondent who presented a paper at a medical humanities–related workshop gave an unconditional "YES." The other two responses suggest that at present such courses or workshops are not offered at those institutions of current

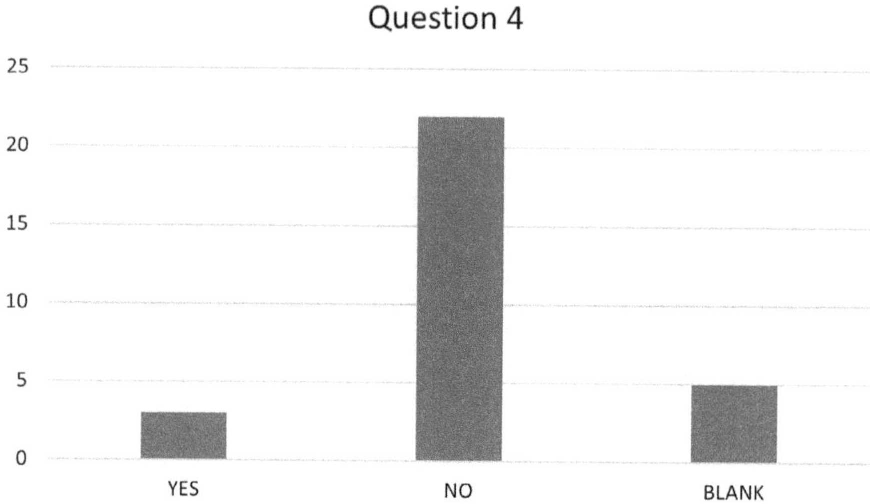

Figure 4.4. Question 4 Responses
Source: Konstantin Starikov

employment. One respondent indicated that s/he taught at Northwestern University Medical School. The other respondent simply provided his/her geographic locations such as Illinois, Washington University in St. Louis, and a Chekhov conference at Colby College funded by the NEH. It was not clear if these were courses or professional workshops and presentations.

Out of twenty-two "NO" responses only three contained comments. One respondent observed that as a result of student interest in hospital interpreting and opportunities to work with Russian-speaking patients the Slavic department offers a language course in Medical Russian. This course is open to medical students. Does this mean that such courses should not be offered at institutions that do not have a medical school? One of the responders implied that this is the case, although the existence of pre-med and pre-health programs allowed him/her to work closely with pre-med advisors to finalize the course syllabus. Another respondent also mentioned that many pre-med students that plan to enroll in medical schools take a course on Chekhov.

Q5

In this question respondents were asked to list five stories by Chekhov which, in their opinion, were the most relevant when teaching topics related to medical humanities. The design of the survey encouraged respondents to list five short stories but did not exclude those who listed less than five stories or other genres (one respondent included in his/her answer Chekhov's non-fiction work *The Island of Sakhalin* and two respondents referenced medical themes in the plays *Uncle Vanya* and *The Cherry Orchard*). Eight respondents did not answer this question. Due to variations translations of Chekhov's titles into English, I have normalized the answers and summarized the frequency of occurrence in the histogram below.

The most frequently occurring short story is "Ward No. 6." Inclusion of this story in a course related to medical humanities appeared self-evident to many respondents, as illustrated by one parenthetical comments ("obviously") and an adjective ("obvious") in another comment: "The most obvious is 'Ward No. 6,' about a medical doctor who ends up in his own mental ward . . ." Another indicator that "Ward No. 6," one of Chekhov's most read stories, occurred immediately to respondents is the order in which they listed the short stories. Out of sixteen respondents who included "Ward No. 6," ten respondents prioritized it over the other stories. It is interesting that among the six respondents who did not chose "Ward No. 6," the most frequently occurring titles in their answers were "Aniuta," "The Black Monk," and "A Boring Story." These stories also reflect the frequency of occurrence in other respondents' answers. "Aniuta" falls into the second category of most frequently listed works (8–9 times; "A Case History" 9, "Aniuta" 8, "An Attack of Nerves" 8). Both "The Black Monk" and "A Boring Story" are the third most frequently mentioned titles in addition to "Sleepy" (6 times).

By comparison, the short story "Misery," which is commonly taught in medical humanities courses by instructors with MD credentials, was not selected by Slavic scholars in our survey. Although it was difficult to assess the scope of the popularity of this and other short stories among medical humanists due to a lack of comprehensive open access databases of syllabi in the field of medical humanities, my review of syllabi using a Google search engine, browsing the NYU Literature and Medicine Database syllabi section, and searching the Open Syllabus Project website identified the following Chekhov short stories as the top five: "Ward No. 6," "Misery," "An Attack of Nerves," "Enemies," "A Case History," and the sixth (each occurring once) "The Black Monk"/"A Boring Story"/"Rothschild's Fiddle"/"An Awkward Business"/"Kashtanka."

The respondents' comments have also provided additional information about the thematic categorization of these stories in the context of teaching medical humanities. One respondent wrote:

> The most obvious is "Ward No. Six," about a medical doctor who ends up in his own mental ward, but "The Darling" and "Man in a Case" would be useful in studying personality disorders, *Uncle Vanya* and *The Cherry Orchard* for the perils of burn-out among physicians (not stories, I know, but especially in *Vanya*, doctors have key roles). "The Student" on how this dehumanization

begins in medical school, "House with the Mansard" for the debate on the very utility of medical care in a society where the poor are hobbled by much more than ill health, "The Name-Day Party," for an amazing depiction of late-term pregnancy and a harrowing miscarriage.

Other themes that were mentioned in the comments are: death, disease, the history of medicine, doctor-patient relationships, mental health, spiritual health, and the practice of medicine in nineteenth century Russia. It was interesting to learn that none of the respondents used the word "empathy," and the word "compassion" occurred only once in a comment to Question 6. According to the thematic categorization on the syllabi, only two instructors chose "Misery" as a short story, which, in their opinion, was relevant to the topic of compassion and empathy, since it was listed under "Compassion, Empathy and Illness" and "Poverty: Justice, Fairness and Compassion." In the other three instances, the instructors assigned the reading of "Misery" under the session topics "On Doctoring," "Doctor-Patient Relationships," and "Patients, Families and Their Suffering." The other thematic rubrics for Chekhov's short stories are "Difficult Encounter," "Rewards and Challenges of Clinical Practice," "Conflicts and Perplexities in the Workplace," "Mental Health," "Literature Medicine and the Privacy of Suffering," and "Class, Power and Storytelling."

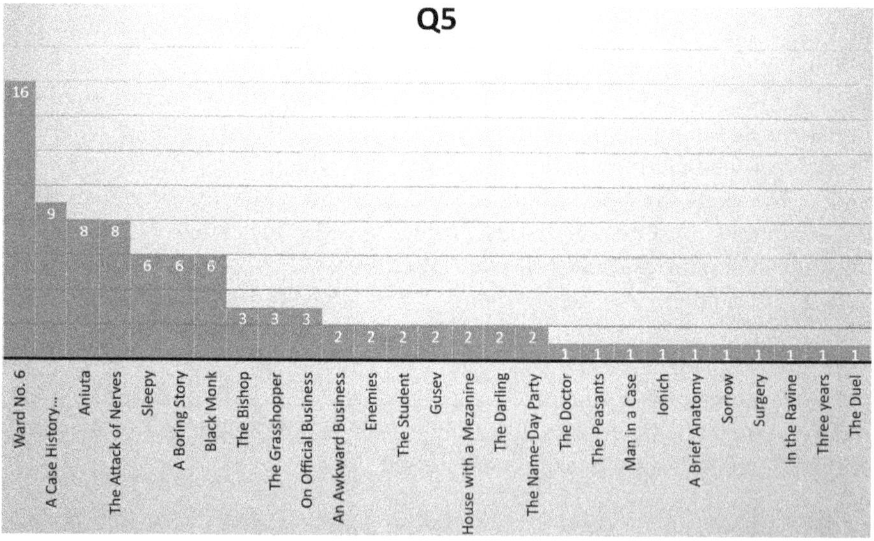

Figure 4.5. Question 5 Responses
Source: Konstantin Starikov

Q6

Rather than asking respondents to evaluate a statement using a Lickert scale, I found it more informative to gauge the respondent's emotional response to a general question. As a result, five respondents underscored their enthusiasm about the idea of Slavic scholars playing a more prominent role in medical education. This observation is inferred from the use of the exclamation point, such as "Yes!" and "Sure!" In other responses one can discern strong agreement but no indication of emotion (i.e., "Absolutely," "Yes—front and center"). Three respondents agreed without any indication of strong agreement ("Yes," "Sure"). Ten respondents provided an affirmative conditional statement implying a lack of interest or indifference ("If they want"), a neutral position ("If individual scholars should so wish, they would have no opposition from me"), lack of interest of teaching in the field of medical humanities ("This is certainly an interesting idea. I support it in general but am unlikely to teach anything along these lines"), lack of experience, opinion, or reflection ("I haven't done any medical humanities, but I suppose Slavic scholars could do it as well as other humanists. Otherwise, I haven't thought about it," "Tentative yes, but I have not put much thought into the issue").

The following comments explain the reasoning of those respondents who support the idea of Slavic scholars participating in medical education. One thinks that "medical humanities is an important and growing field, and for those Slavists who are interested in it, yes, I think we can play a role." It is noteworthy that this comment was made by a faculty member whose institution does not have a medical humanities program or a medical school. Another faculty member at a different institution with a medical humanities program and a medical school emphasized that major Russian writers pay "exceptional attention" to the human condition.

Some respondents expressed the point of view that pre-med students and doctors would benefit from reading Russian literature on medical and non-medical topics either taught individually or co-taught by a literary scholar and a medical professional ("Yes, I think that to be a good doctor, a medical student must read and understand literature as part of his training, for it is only through literature that one can grasp the most elusive thing of all—the human psyche"; "Yes. It would be an excellent initiative to design and offer courses in medical humanities co-taught by a literary scholar and a medical professional. I have been thinking about pursuing such a teaching project at X").

Other respondents shared the opinion that literary scholars in general, not just Slavic literary scholars, could teach about empathy and compassion to the medical community. This opinion was shared even among those who gave an ambivalent answer ("As much as any scholar") or a negative answer ("Not necessarily. Literary scholars are not trained to do this. I do agree that some fine literature can teach medical professionals about the human condition and about compassion. This is the role of literature in society. And doctors, as treaters of human ailments, are advised to learn from good literature").

Two responses demonstrated uncertainty regarding the success of Slavic scholars in playing a role in medical education. As mentioned previously, one respondent felt that the administrative challenges are unsurmountable, which implies a pessimistic albeit sympathetic point of view ("Probably. It can be difficult to get up the energy to tackle the bureaucratic barriers"). The other respondent perhaps displayed more optimism by advocating direct action ("Certainly, but it will be up to us to open up such a space for our work: nobody will offer it to us").

Among the respondents who answered "NO" there were two respondents, both specialists in Chekhov, who disagreed with the formulation of the question. For example, one respondent said: "Not sure what this question means. Does medical education need Slavists in particular? Literature, yes; Russian literature, not necessarily. Or should Slavic literary scholars be obligated to be involved in medical education? Of course not." A second respondent disagreed with the question as formulated for the following reasons: "The question is strangely put, and given the way it is put, I would have to answer, no not as a rule. Certainly, there should be a place for Slavic literary scholars with interest and competence in medical humanities (narrative medicine, forensic literary scholarship, literature and psychology, etc.) in medical

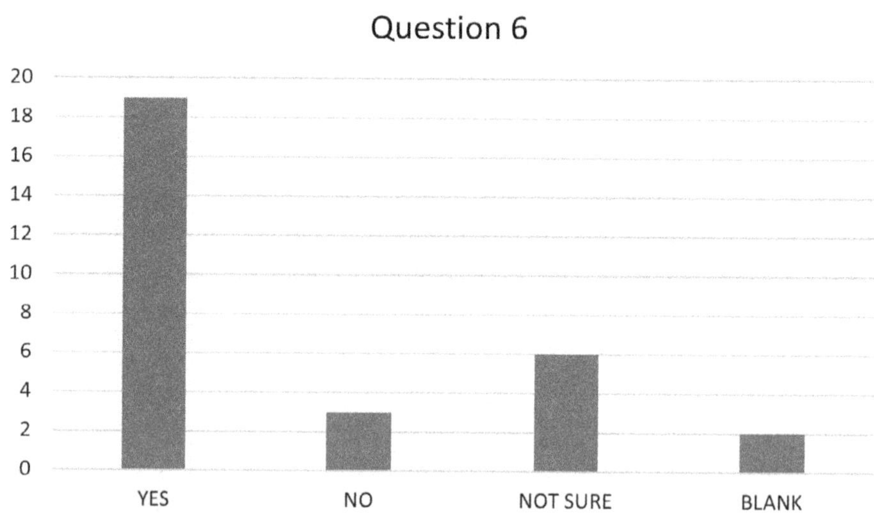

Figure 4.6. Question 6 Responses
Source: Konstantin Starikov

humanities programs. And why shouldn't they be included among other humanists teaching in programs of medical education? There are plenty of materials available in translation for courses focused on Russia for students without Russian, and the history of medicine in Russia is quite interesting and different from ours in many ways. Of course, many Slavic scholars work at institutions in locations where there aren't medical or nursing schools. One doesn't need to be involved in medical education to pursue one's research interest in medical humanities or to incorporate it into courses."

It is also noteworthy that only a single respondent expressed concern about Slavic literary scholars teaching medical students without any special training. This is noteworthy because it shows that the issue of training is not a major impediment and that those faculty who already teach courses which include themes of medical humanities would feel comfortable in participating in a medical humanities program.

DISCUSSION

The response of the survey was 50 percent (30 out of n=60 faculty affiliated with Slavic departments). More than half of the respondents answered that either they don't have a medical humanities program at their institution (n=13 or 43.3%) or they are uncertain if it exists (n=6 or 20%). Only a little over a quarter of respondents (n=8 or 26.7%) have a medical humanities program at their institution. A third of respondents (n=10 or 33.3%) have taught undergraduate courses which incorporated Slavic literary texts relevant to the field of medical humanities. Twenty percent of respondents (n=6 or 20%) incorporated Slavic literary texts in a graduate-level course or workshop. The majority of respondents have never taught a course or a workshop to medical students or hospital staff which incorporated Slavic literary texts relevant to the study of medical humanities. Only 10 percent (n=3 or 10%) said that they have taught medical students or hospital staff.

Sixty-three percent of respondents (n=19 or 63.3%) supported the idea of Slavic literary scholars taking a role in medical education. Twenty percent of faculty (n=6 or 20%) expressed uncertainty, and 10 percent (n=3 or 10%) said "no" because of disagreement with the formulation of the question or lack of proper training. In their comments, one can discern a point of view which recognizes the value of medical humanities programs and the role that literature can play in this context.

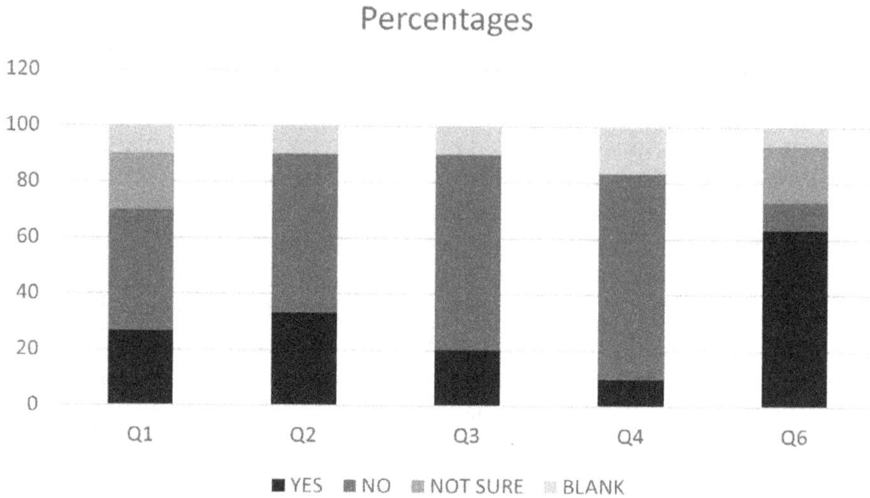

Figure 4.7. Summary of Results for Q1–Q4 and Q6
Source: Konstantin Starikov

Due to a lack of a comprehensive database or an open access repository of syllabi in the field of Slavic studies, or for that matter in the field of medical humanities, it is difficult to say how accurate the representation of suggested Chekhov stories is in relation to actual reading lists. For further analysis, one could compare the list of suggested primary sources (i.e., short stories) provided by Cathy Popkin in the appendix to her essay "Chekhov and the Medical Humanities"[8] and the top five Chekhov stories suggested by the respondents:

Table 4.1. Question 5 Responses

Chekhov Story	*Survey Results*	*Popkin's Recommended List*
"A Boring Story"	Yes	No
"A Case History" ("A Medical Case")	Yes (top 5)	Yes
"A Nervous Breakdown" ("An Attack of Nerves")	Yes (top 5)	Yes
"Aniuta"	Yes (top 5)	Yes
"Enemies"	Yes	Yes
"Sleepy"	Yes (top 5)	No
"The Student"	Yes	Yes
"Rothschild's Fiddle"	No	Yes
"Ward No. 6"	Yes (top 5)	Yes

The frequency of occurrence of titles in the survey may provide additional information about the relevance of Chekhov stories in the context of teaching medical humanities. "Ward No. 6" was the top choice among the respondents. Although this short story is usually incorporated into course modules on issues such as mental health, it could also be of additional value to a medical student or a practicing physician through the pairing of its stylistic analysis with another popular Russian literary text often taught in medical humanities courses, Tolstoy's *The Death of Ivan Ilych*. These stories may help medical students to acquire competency in the analyzing and interpreting a narrative point of view. Michael Finke attributes the shift in narrative point of view in "Ward No. 6" and other Chekhov stories to his stylistic experimentations after his own near-death experience and Tolstoy's artistic influence. Hence, a traditional stylistic analysis in which the Slavic literary scholar has been trained can enhance pragmatic discussions about subjectivity in the experience of illness.

The shift in narrative strategy in Chekhov's stories demonstrates mastery of a narrative which teaches how to discern empathy and compassion in the other.[9] As Finke correctly stipulated, Chekhov's affiliation with two professions, that of a writer and a doctor, is a two-way street.[10] This is evident in Chekhov's own proposed pedagogical approach to teaching first-year medical students by seeking to engage them with the subjective experience of a patient.[11] Since medical practitioners rely on narrative practices and patients' stories when treating a disease, the skills of engagement based on ethical reasoning, empathy, and compassion are acquired best through the reconstruction of subjectivity in a literary text. As a writer whose prose reflected his medical training, Chekhov is not simply of interest to medical students because of the plethora of medical themes in his fiction but also as a doctor whose creative writing can become a lifelong companion in the art of diagnosis to a practicing physician.

Of course, as some respondents mentioned, the issues of training, expertise, academic interests, and administrative hurdles may hinder a Slavic scholar from participating in a medical humanities program. There are nearly 150 medical schools in the US and Canada that offer medical, nursing, and public health programs.[12] About two-thirds of medical schools have a medical humanities program. Some Slavic scholars work at institutions which do not have a medical school or a medical humanities program, but most academic institutions—even those that are not affiliated with a hospital or do not have a medical community—do have pre-med and other health-related programs.

How well would a Slavic scholar fit in a medical humanities program? Since it is an interdisciplinary field which already consists of humanists from English Literature, Comparative Literatures, Theater, Dance, and other liberal arts departments, I would argue that a Slavic literary scholar would receive a warm welcome. Certainly, there may be resistance from doctors who enjoy teaching and find it rewarding to use literary texts on a personal and professional level. Many medical staff volunteer their time to teach medical humanities because they discover that this new experience offers them a unique opportunity to get to know their third and fourth students better outside of a clinical setting which affords little time for philosophical conversations. But others may find that the opportunity to co-teach with a humanist or even observe how a literary analysis is done by a scholar specializing in Chekhov, Bulgakov, or Tolstoy will benefit everyone as they, too, still can use this experience when teaching a class or a workshop individually.

The kinds of questions then that a Slavic scholar could consider are: what is my incentive for teaching literature to medical students? If my institution has a medical school or a medical humanities program how will my department view my initiative of co-teaching a course with a medical professional? How will a medical student benefit from my humanistic training of teaching Chekhov, Bulgakov, or Tolstoy? In my view, it is not simply a matter of opportunity to seek another academic venue for teaching Russian literature when enrollments in Russian literature and language courses are on the decline. It, too, is a two-way street because a Slavic scholar can make a difference in the quality of healthcare by educating medical students about empathy and compassion. Cathy Popkin's and Michael Finke's emphasis that Chekhov's literary prose is already taught in the context of medical humanities is a convincing argument that many Slavic literary scholars are already in the business of medical humanities. That most of the surveyed scholars think that it is a good idea to seek a more prominent role in medical education is a positive sign of bridging the field of medical humanities with Slavic studies.

Bringing Slavic literature into medical education could also help those medical communities that encounter patients from Eastern Europe. Medical students and doctors alike will be able identify the cultural elements of local East European communities. For example, St. Elizabeth's Medical Center in Boston created a Russian-American Institute of Medicine that treats Russian-speaking patients from Russia and the former Soviet Union. The United States and Canada are also home to Ukrainian, Polish, and other Slavic diaspora communities. For this reason, the survey questions asked about *Slavic* literary texts. All responses, as expected, were focused on Russian authors, except for one respondent who described an ongoing project of translating an account of burning vampires alive in Ukraine during a cholera epidemic by the Ukrainian poet Ivan Franko (1856–1916)

CONCLUSION

One of many examples in which literature, and Russian literature in particular, is used as a major force that can help create narratives to interpret illness and assign meaning to life is evident from searching the medical journals indexed in MEDLINE, EMBASE, and CINAHL. As recently as January 2017, the *Lancet* journal published a letter by two faculty members, Andrea Rodriguez-Prat, Department of Humanities, and Cristina Monforte-Royo, Department of Nursing, School of Medicine and Health Sciences at the Universitat Internacional de Catalunya, Barcelona, in which they write: "Humanities could help find the forgotten words patients might need to hear for them to create their own stories. They could give health professionals the tools to be not only Virgils, but Odysseuses looking for their origin, or *Ivan Ilyches* [K.S.] unveiling gestures of care and comprehension on the deathbed."[13]

Chekhov's Ragins and Astrovs, too, are of great interest to doctors in English-speaking medical settings.[14] In 2008, the editorial board of the *Journal of Public Health* inaugurated a regular feature titled "Chekhov's Corner," which focuses on the intersection of the humanities with public health practice.[15] One of the contributors to Chekhov's Corner used the following explanation to underscore the importance of broadening the medical imagination of students and junior doctors by using literary texts:

> As an academic internist, I teach medical students and junior doctors in both the inpatient and outpatient settings. I have often been disappointed in how easily the house staff lose the trees for the forest. Too often, they take a "population" approach to their patients, though not exactly in the public health sense, more in a category approach: Chest pain patient = telemetry, serial enzymes, echo, stress. Pneumonia patient = X-ray, IV ceftriaxone plus azithro. Altered mental status patient = CT, LP, pan-culture, broad-spectrum antibiotics.
>
> A few years ago I began to supplement rounds with readings from classic literature or our own Bellevue Literary Review. I always chose stories, essays, or poems that specifically highlighted the individual. I wanted to use literature's greatest strength—the uniqueness of the protagonist—to remind junior doctors that because each patient's chest pain occurs in a different life that each chest-pain story is, by definition, exceptional.[16]

Given the growing realization of the benefits of medical humanities in the medical community it is paramount that Slavic scholars are exposed to the mission of the medical humanists. Further investigations of the interactions between Slavic scholars and the medical professionals are desirable in order to gauge how well Chekhov scholars, for instance, are familiar with the publications about Chekhov in medical literature, medical schools, or public health and nursing programs. How many Chekhov scholars are currently involved in contributing to the advancement of medical humanities programs at their institutions? Do they submit articles to medical journals?

It is important that Slavic scholars develop a sense of collegiality with the medical community even if they are not interested in co-teaching or working directly with them. Slavic librarians may also find themselves in the new role of liaison with doctors who are interested in using the expertise of scholars in Slavic departments. Compiling bibliographies of useful readings from medical literature, which is out of the scope of traditional academic reading, and regularly sharing them via a newsletter or an email can be a useful library service. For example, in the "Literature and the Arts in Medical Education" section of the journal *Family Medicine,* contributors summarize literary and artistic works used in medical education, discuss their purpose and goals in using these materials, teaching strategies, methods of evaluations, and offer theoretical views on these teaching tools.[17]

The resistance to introducing literary content into medical education may be expressed both by medical students who often see them as peripheral and irrelevant as well as by specialists in the field.[18] It is therefore recommended to invite medical humanists for workshops and talks designed for Slavic faculty and department administrators which will provide an opportunity to engage Slavic scholars with the mission of medical humanities. In his article "The Good Doctor: The Literature and Medicine of Anton Chekhov (and Others)," Dr. Lawrence Schneiderman recollected a failed conversation he had with a Slavic scholar with expertise in Chekhov in 1985:

> In the spring of 1985, I posted a notice on the medical students' bulletin board announcing a new elective course, "The Good Doctor: The Literature and Medicine of Anton Chekhov." It was a presumptuous announcement, since I had never taught a literature course and had never even participated in a book discussion group. Naturally, I looked for experienced colleagues to help me out. My first contact was not encouraging. A professor with expertise in Chekhov bluntly refused to have anything to do with me. "I don't want a doctor who knows Chekhov, I want a doctor who knows how to take out my appendix." Fortunately, I was able to locate two more agreeable colleagues from literature and theatre.[19]

With the growing acceptance of medical humanities courses in US and Canadian medical schools the anecdotal gap between MDs and PhDs may not be as stark today. Even though there are still questions and even doubts about the efficacy of medical humanities programs, the proliferation of medical humanities as an academic field reflects the growing acceptance of the new role of medical humanities educators with a variety of degrees, expertise, and scholarly interests. Many pioneers in the humanities were and continue to be at the crossroads of the humanities and medicine, similar in experience to Chekhov, who practiced both medicine and literature.

The results of this survey show that there is interest among Slavic scholars who are familiar with medical humanities and genuine support for the idea of Slavic scholars becoming more involved with medical humanities. This is a point of view shared even by some Slavic scholars who are unlikely to collaborate with the medical community in the future. The survey data also supports my original hypothesis that Slavic scholars teach literary texts with medical themes or topics relevant to the field of medical humanities mainly in their home departments, with almost no interaction with medical students or medical staff.

Why would medical faculty be interested in working with a literary scholar? After all, medical students are not expected to excel in literary analysis. The success of a medical humanities program may depend on the level of expertise of the literary scholars in order to keep these programs interesting and intellectually engaged from the perspective of medical students. Co-teaching arrangements by both physicians and literary scholars are a vital part of a long tradition to understand one another.[20] If a medical humanities program does not exist at one's institution, as the majority of respondents indicated in the survey, there are opportunities for Slavic scholars interested in medical humanities to team up with other humanities faculty and members of the medical community in the area (for example, hospitals and health centers if a university or college does not have a medical school) to conceive of a collaborative approach and submit a proposal as a cohesive group. As an example, the HumMed program at Lund University in Sweden was created by a small team consisting of two humanities faculty and four medical faculty, supported by the university administration.[21]

In summary, a Slavic scholar with a specialization in Chekhov or Bulgakov can make a meaningful and lasting contribution to medical education. The field of medical humanities is in need of faculty in Slavic departments who have experience teaching Tolstoy, Alexander Solzhenitsyn (1918–2008), and other authors who were not doctors but employed literature to inculcate empathy and portray the protagonist as a unique individual. Upon entering the world of clinical discourse in culturally diverse medical environments, medical students will also better appreciate the narrative of illness if they are exposed in their medical humanities courses to a range of multilingual literary texts, including the works in translation of East European writers.

NOTES

1. Cleveland Clinic, "Medical Humanities Accent the Human Touch," *Alumni Connection*, vol. 21, no. 2, 2011: 1–7, 6.

2. Charon, Rita, et al., *The Principles and Practice of Narrative Medicine*, Oxford: Oxford University Press, 2017.

3. Chekhov, Anton, *Letters of Anton Chekhov to His Family and Friends* (Trans. Garnett, C.), Project Gutenberg, http://gutenberg.org/files/6408/6408-h/6408-h.htm#link2H_4_004.

4. Corso, Thomas, "Designing a Literature and Medicine Course for the Physician Assistant Studies Curriculum," *The Journal of Physician Assistant Education*, vol. 12, no. 3, 2001: 181–186.

5. Pellegrino, Edmund D., *Humanism and the Physician*, Knoxville: University of Tennessee Press, 1979, 9.

6. Peschel, Enid Rhodes, *Medicine and Literature*, New York: N. Watson Academic Publications, 1980, 2.

7. Karlinsky, S. *Letters of Anton Chekhov* (Trans. Heim, H.), New York: Harper & Row, 1972, 367.

8. Finke, Michael C., and Michael Holquist, *Approaches to Teaching the Works of Anton Chekhov*, New York: The Modern Language Association of America, 2016, 151.

9. Charon, Rita, *Narrative Medicine: Honoring the Stories of Illness*, Oxford: Oxford University Press, 2006, 118.

10. Finke and Holquist, *Approaches to Teaching the Works of Anton Chekhov,* 62.

11. For more see Rossolimo, G. I., "Vospominaniia o Chekhove," in *Chekhov v vospominaniiakh sovremennikov*, edited by N. Gitovich, Moscow: Khudozh. lit-ra, 1986: 428–438.

12. Crawford, Paul, et al., *Health Humanities*, New York: Palgrave, 2015, 16.

13. Rodríguez-Prat, Andrea, and Cristina Monforte-Royo, "25 Years after Intoxicated by My Illness: Challenges for Medical Humanities," *The Lancet*, vol. 389, no. 10066, Jan. 2017: 249–250.

14. For more see Crommelynck, Isabelle, "Doctor Chekhov's Doctors," *Frontiers of Neurology and Neuroscience*, vol. 31, 2013: 236–244.

15. For more see Leung, G. M., "Musings on Chekhov," *Journal of Public Health* (Oxford, England), vol. 30, no. 2, 2008: 117–118.

16. Ofri, Danielle, "Public Health and the Muse," *Journal of Public Health* (Oxford, England), vol. 30, no. 2, June 2008: 205–208, 205.

17. Schneiderman, L.J., "The Good Doctor: The Literature and Medicine of Anton Chekhov (and Others)," *Family Medicine*, edited by Johanna Shapiro, vol. 33, no. 1, Jan. 2001: 11–13, 11.

18. Oyebode, Femi, and Victoria Tischler, "Applying Narrative to Medical Education," in *Narrative Matters in Medical Contexts across Disciplines*, edited by Franziska Gygax and Miriam Locher, Amsterdam: John Benjamins Publishing Company, 2015: 183–206, 203.

19. Schneiderman, "The Good Doctor: The Literature and Medicine of Anton Chekhov (and Others)," 11.

20. For more see Hunter, K. M., et al., "The Study of Literature in Medical Education," *Academic Medicine: Journal of the Association of American Medical Colleges*, vol. 70, no. 9, Sept. 1995: 787–794.

21. Wachtler, Caroline, et al., "Humanities for Medical Students? A Qualitative Study of a Medical Humanities Curriculum in a Medical School Program," *BMC Medical Education*, vol. 6, Mar. 2006: 16, 4.

WORKS CITED

Charon, Rita. *Narrative Medicine: Honoring the Stories of Illness*. Oxford: Oxford University Press, 2006.

Charon, Rita, et al. *The Principles and Practice of Narrative Medicine*. Oxford: Oxford University Press, 2017.

Chekhov, Anton. *Letters of Anton Chekhov to His Family and Friends*. (Trans. Garnett, C.) Project Gutenberg, http://gutenberg.org/files/6408/6408-h/6408-h.htm#link2H_4_004.

Cleveland Clinic. "Medical Humanities Accent the Human Touch." *Alumni Connection*, vol. 21, no. 2, 2011: 1–7.

Corso, Thomas. "Designing a Literature and Medicine Course for the Physician Assistant Studies Curriculum." *The Journal of Physician Assistant Education*, vol. 12, no. 3, 2001: 181–186.

Crawford, Paul, et al. *Health Humanities*. New York: Palgrave, 2015.

Crommelynck, Isabelle. "Doctor Chekhov's Doctors." *Frontiers of Neurology and Neuroscience*, vol. 31, 2013: 236–244.

Finke, Michael C., and Michael Holquist. *Approaches to Teaching the Works of Anton Chekhov*. New York: The Modern Language Association of America, 2016.

Hunter, K. M., et al. "The Study of Literature in Medical Education." *Academic Medicine: Journal of the Association of American Medical Colleges*, vol. 70, no. 9, Sept. 1995: 787–794.

Karlinsky, S. *Letters of Anton Chekhov*. (Trans. Heim, H.) New York: Harper & Row, 1972.

Leung, G. M. "Musings on Chekhov." *Journal of Public Health* (Oxford, England), vol. 30, no. 2, 2008: 117–118.

Ofri, Danielle. "Public Health and the Muse." *Journal of Public Health* (Oxford, England), vol. 30, no. 2, June 2008: 205–208.

Oyebode, Femi, and Victoria Tischler. "Applying Narrative to Medical Education." In *Narrative Matters in Medical Contexts across Disciplines*, edited by Franziska Gygax and Miriam Locher. Amsterdam: John Benjamins Publishing Company, 2015: 183–206.

Pellegrino, Edmund D. *Humanism and the Physician*. Knoxville: University of Tennessee Press, 1979.

Peschel, Enid Rhodes. *Medicine and Literature*. New York: N. Watson Academic Publications, 1980.

Rodríguez-Prat, Andrea, and Cristina Monforte-Royo. "25 Years after Intoxicated by My Illness: Challenges for Medical Humanities." *The Lancet*, vol. 389, no. 10066, Jan. 2017: 249–250.

Rossolimo, G.I. "Vospominaniia o Chekhove." In *Chekhov v vospominaniiakh sovremennikov*, edited by N. Gitovich, Moscow: Khudozh. lit-ra, 1986: 428–438.

Schneiderman, L.J. "The Good Doctor: The Literature and Medicine of Anton Chekhov (and Others)." *Family Medicine*, edited by Johanna Shapiro, vol. 33, no. 1, Jan. 2001: 11–13.

Self, Donnie J., editor. *The Role of the Humanities in Medical Education*. Bio-Medical Ethics Program, Eastern Virginia Medical School, 1978.

Snow, C.P. *The Two Cultures and the Scientific Revolution*. Cambridge: Cambridge University Press, 1961.

Wachtler, Caroline, et al. "Humanities for Medical Students? A Qualitative Study of a Medical Humanities Curriculum in a Medical School Program." *BMC Medical Education*, vol. 6, Mar. 2006: 16.

Part II

MEDICAL ENCOUNTERS IN LITERATURE AND CULTURE

Chapter Five

Pauline Tarnowsky and the Russian Influence on Cesare Lombroso's *Criminal Woman*

Frederick H. White

In 1893, Cesare Lombroso (1835–1909) and Guglielmo Ferrero (1871–1942) co-authored *Criminal Woman, the Prostitute and the Normal Woman* (*La donna delinquente, la prostituta e la donna normale*), which attempted to establish a typology of female criminals. Specific attention was given to physical signs of "primitiveness" that indicated a reduced maternal sense in these women. Lombroso and Ferrero expected ideal femininity in their subjects, designated as normal, with any anomaly classified as an indication of sexual deviance and social dangerousness. Combining the evolutionary theories of Charles Darwin (1809–1882) with the science of statistics, Lombroso and Ferrero studied the criminal, rather than the crime.

At the end of the nineteenth century, Russian intellectuals were particularly interested in this new approach and embraced the new methods of criminal anthropology as a way to bring science into the courtroom. Paradoxically, it was the research of the Russian physician Praskov'ia Tarnovskaia (1848–1910) that informed Lombroso and Ferrero's study on female offenders. In fact, Tarnovskaia's own research on prostitutes and thieves returned to Russia and was more broadly read than Lombroso and Fererro's supposedly groundbreaking study *Criminal Woman*. As a result, Sharon A. Kowalsky has argued that "despite the interest, no serious attempt was made before 1893 to develop specific theories that addressed the causes of women's deviance."[1]

In this chapter, I will revisit Tarnovskaia's research in order to suggest that the Russian physician had a greater influence on Lombroso's concept of female criminality than has previously been asserted.[2] In so doing, I will show that Tarnovskaia (known as Pauline Tarnowsky outside of Russia) was acknowledged in the West as one of the leading criminal anthropologists and respected for her scholarly work. Finally, although this will not be the main interest of this chapter, I will assert that within the context of the medical humanities, the lasting interest in Tarnovskaia's research may now be the personal histories of many of the female offenders that accompanied these anatomical statistics.[3]

Previously, Lombroso had suggested that physical anomalies of an atavistic origin distinguished male non-criminals from male criminals. According to Lombroso the criminal was a subspecies of man with distinct physical and mental characteristics. Physical signs of atavism were found in the skull, brain, and other parts of the skeleton, muscles, and viscera. These anatomical peculiarities signified that the individual was a "throwback" to earlier primate stages of evolution, a "savage" inclined to violence. The assertion of a criminal subspecies that was predisposed to brutality, amorality, and anarchy seemed to negate the possibility of social rejuvenation. At odds with Lombroso's theory of atavism was the concept of degeneration. Bénédict Augustin Morel (1809–1873) had originally suggested that hereditary traits and environmental factors contributed to the biological material within a family. Arguably, mental illness and behavioral abnormalities were indicative of an anomalous constitution. A compromised nervous system was passed through the generations allowing for the accumulation of moral, mental, and physical disorders, which resulted in the rapid degeneration of a family line. Rather than a born criminal subspecies, degeneration theory offered stable criteria for predicting the hereditary transmission of crime, sickness, and mental disorders from generation to generation.

Daniel Beer has argued that Russian criminologists and psychiatrists responded positively to the theory that the criminal, rather than the crime, should be the focus of legal and medical attention. Many also accepted Lombroso's assertion of a born criminal, while still rejecting the idea that criminality was independent of social factors. The notion that criminals were beyond the reach of societal influence clashed with the Russian intelligentsia's long-held belief that education and material improvement could positively transform members of a society. As a result, Russian scientists turned to degeneration theory in place of Lombroso's assertion of atavism with the belief that environmental factors acquired over a lifetime could be transmitted from one generation to the next.[4]

Degeneration also seemed to offer an explanation for the problems of a Russian society plagued by a legacy of serfdom, economic backwardness, and social stratification, not to mention endemic crime, public health issues, and numerous crises that had negatively affected the Russian national identity. After all, the notion of social progress and the possibility that Russia was moving in the wrong direction had long been an obsession of the nineteenth century.[5] Alarmingly, industrial modernization seemed to exacerbate further this perceived social and moral regression of the entire nation.[6] Gratefully, science offered an explanation for this national problem and the newest medical science, psychiatry, was needed in order to discover a remedy that might lead to national regeneration.

Following the establishment of the first independent department of psychiatry at the Imperial Medical-Surgical Academy in 1860, the most promising students were given stipends to complete their studies in European laboratories and clinics with eminent scientists such as Jacques-Joseph Moreau (1804–1884) and Jean-Martin Charcot (1823–1893). At the time, Lombroso's *Criminal Man* (*L'uomo delinquente*, 1876; second edition 1878; French edition 1887; German edition 1889; fifth and final edition 1896–1897) was highly influential. Originally this book consisted of one volume and 225 pages but was four volumes and over 2,000 pages in its final edition. Daniel G. Horn has noted that in this final version *Criminal Man* was a heterogeneous text full of contradictions, "organized by an ambition to build a totalizing science of criminal man."[7] Maybe exactly for this reason, Lombroso's theory of the born criminal dominated the Russian scientific discourse.

Issak Orshanskii (1851–1923) completed his dissertation in St. Petersburg in 1876 and then spent a year and a half studying nervous disorders in Berlin, Leipzig, and Paris, before becoming a professor of psychiatry at Kharkov University. Orshanskii supported the scientific ideas of Lombroso, Bénédict Augustin Morel, and Valentin Magnan (1835–1916) in publications such as *Our Criminals and the Studies of Lombroso* (*Nashi prestupniki i uchenie Lombrozo*, 1890) and *The Role of Heredity in the Transfer of Illness* (*Rol' nasledstvennosti v peredache boleznei*, 1894).[8] Nikolai Bazhenov (1856–1923) worked with Charcot and Magnan in Europe where he studied the skulls and busts of criminals. Eventually, Bazhenov became medical director of the Moscow City Psychiatric Hospital.[9] At Kharkov University, Pavel Kovalevskii (1849–1923), an ardent Lombroso disciple, was editor of the journal *Archive of Psychiatry, Neurology, and Forensic Psychopathology* (*Arkhiv psikhiatrii, neirologii, i sudebnoi psikhopatologii*, 1883–1899). He conducted psychological and anatomical research on famous people and studied the effects of syphilis on the nervous system.[10] Vladimir Bekhterev (1857–1927) was head of psychiatry at the University of Kazan and editor of *The Herald of Psychology, Criminal Anthropology and Hypnosis* (*Vestnik psikhologii, kriminal'noi antropologii, i gipnoza*, 1904–1919; later *Hypnosis* was replaced by *Pediatrics*).[11] These leading Russian psychiatrists were committed to addressing the devolution of Russian society, which seemed to be a demonstrable, scientific fact.[12]

Bekhterev, Dmitrii Dril' (1846–1910), Vladimir Chizh (1855–1922), Tarnovskaia, and Veniamin Tarnovskii (1837–1906) were supporters of Lombroso and regular attendees at the *International Congresses of Criminal*

Anthropology. By the beginning of the twentieth century, Dril' was one of the leading Russian specialists on correctional institutions for juveniles.[13] He had published an influential study on young criminals (1884–88) and a detailed history of criminal anthropology (1895).[14] Chizh graduated from the Medical-Surgical Academy in 1878 and eventually became an assistant physician at a prison hospital in 1881 where he began to study the connection between crime and insanity. He combined Lombroso's theory of the born criminal with research on moral insanity to explain the perceived moral and mental degeneration of the prison population.[15] Tarnovskaia was the daughter of the former director of the St. Petersburg Academy of Military Medicine, Nikolai Kozlov, and the wife of the venereologist Veniamin Tarnovskii.

Both Tarnovskaia and her husband specialized in the areas of prostitution and sexual perversion; both were internationally recognized as experts on criminal anthropology. However, husband and wife had very different responses to the issue. Tarnovskii advocated for administrative measures to regulate prostitution, while Tarnovskaia believed in social reform, despite the fact that both were advocates of Lombroso's theories on the born criminal.[16] Tarnovskaia was less deterministic than Lombroso when it came to the theory of atavism. She held that social issues played a substantial role in criminal behavior and supported social rejuvenation over judicial repression. Kowalsky has stated that Tarnovskaia's research was part of a "promotion of social hygiene and social welfare." She believed that "criminal anthropology would elucidate the causes of crime and help to develop measures for prevention, particularly by identifying those naturally predisposed to criminal activity, that is, born criminals."[17] For Russian researchers, there was a belief that social forces contributed to the origins of criminality, but there was no uniform agreement on the responsibility of the government or society to address social issues exacerbated by rapid industrialization.[18]

At the second *International Congress of Criminal Anthropology* (1889) held in Paris, French criminologists attacked Lombroso's theory of the born criminal. Alessandre Lacassagne (1843–1924) and Léonce Manouvrier (1850–1927) considered social issues more important than biological factors in determining criminal behavior. Lacassagne thought that the Italian school had exaggerated their claims of atavism, ignoring the social environment. Manouvrier argued that there were no physical differences between honest men and criminals.[19] Daniel Pick has described how the French Lamarckian tradition of inheritance and environmental agency contrasted with the Italian reliance on Darwin's theory of struggle, selection, and elimination. This difference of interpretation was informed by their disparate national histories, which contributed to their scientific dispute. Morel's theories were informed by successive French revolutions, while Lombroso was concerned with the recalcitrance of certain anti-social (criminal) families in Italy. Both French and Italian criminology rejected the early-nineteenth-century insistence that every individual was a legal subject and that the punishment should fit the crime.[20] According to Irina Sirotkina, Russian delegates followed this debate closely and most Russian researchers joined the French contingent against Lombroso's theory of atavism.[21] Zygmunt Ronald Bialkowski has argued that Russian medical researchers "wanted the authoritative trappings of Lombrosianism without the responsibility for his methodology."[22]

As a response to these attacks made at the second congress, Lombroso began a new project on criminal women. He was well acquainted with Tarnovskaia's research and Lombroso would rely heavily on her *An Anthropological Study of Prostitutes and Female Thieves* (*Étude anthropométrique sur les prostituées et les voleuses*, 1889) in organizing his own project.[23] In fact, Lombroso would employ similar methods and reach the same conclusions as his Russian colleague. Notably, Sander Gilman has emphatically stated that Lombroso "repeated word for word" Tarnovskaia's research in *Criminal Woman.* "Lombroso accepts all of Tarnowsky's perceptions of the prostitute," adding only one additional subtext, that of the Hottentot.[24] Just as important, Tarnovskaia's use of a control group and the discussion of social factors might have influenced Lombroso as both appeared for the first time in his research on female offenders. It is reasonable to imagine that the intellectual discourse between Lombroso and Tarnovskaia helped both to advance their research methodology, especially after such a strongly negative reaction from the French school.

In *An Anthropological Study of Prostitutes and Female Thieves*, Tarnovskaia provided a detailed physiognomy of 150 St. Petersburg prostitutes and 100 repeat offenders. These women were compared to an equal number of "honest" women of the same age, race, and from the same geographical areas.[25] Notably, she selected 100 illiterate peasants and 50 educated women from St. Petersburg as a control group of normal women. Tarnovskaia established a triangular relationship between the prostitute, female criminal, and normal woman in order to create a criterion for criminality. According to Tarnovskaia, Morel's *On the Formation of Type in Degenerated Varieties* (*De la formation du type dans les variétés dégénérées*, 1865) was the starting point for her study with a particular interest in the hereditary transmission of degenerate traits. This is where Tarnovskaia deviated from Lombroso's theory of atavism. Significantly, Lombroso too would eventually move in a similar scientific direction.[26]

Among the prostitutes, Tarnovskaia was mainly interested in women who had selected prostitution voluntarily and not those who had been forced into the profession by circumstance. Therefore, all of the prostitutes in her study were officially registered and had been living in brothels for at least three years. Pointedly, Tarnovskaia asserted that a woman of sound mind and body would not choose to be a prostitute, therefore the fact that a large number of women willingly chose this profession was compelling and undermined the arguments of philanthropic organizations. Tarnovskaia wished to explore "the moral level of this class of women in order to find out if their psychic state did not agree with some physical deviations and did not translate into signs of degeneration."[27]

As a result, Tarnovskaia described her subjects' weight, hair, and eye color as well as anthropometric measurements of various parts of the body and a record of family background. These were offered to show signs of degeneration with special attention to facial abnormalities. In this research was evident the discipline of statistics that had come to dominate scientific discourse of the time.[28] It was believed that a typology of criminals could be established through scientific measurement that would reveal the anatomy of deviant bodies. A contributing influence in this area was Colonel Nikolai Kozlov, who had supplemented the Bertillion system to establish an anthropometric station for the St. Petersburg police, which eventually became the model for the all-imperial network of similar stations. The Bertillion system was based on five primary measurements (head length; head breadth; length of middle finger; length of left foot; length of forearm—elbow to end of middle finger) as well as hair and eye color, and front and side view photographs, all of which were recorded and kept on a cardboard form. By 1890, it was a mandatory police practice in St. Petersburg to take these measurements. Seven years later, Kozlov's anthropometric station was replicated in Reval (Tallinn), Novgorod, Grodno, Viatka, Vologda, Vitebsk, Yaroslavl, Odessa, Samarkand, Khabarovsk, and Vladivostok. Moscow adopted the practice in 1900.[29] Therefore, Tarnovskaia's own research on female criminals shared obvious parallels with the use the Bertillion system for police investigations.

Not surprisingly, Tarnovskaia argued that there were marked anatomical differences between normal women and prostitutes.[30] Having provided the anthropometric evidence, Tarnovskaia wished to identify "the hereditary influence suffered by prostitutes as well as the signs of degeneration."[31] The stigmata of degeneration once again were concentrated mainly on facial and dental features, as well as visible anomalies of the skull or ears, which were found more often in prostitutes than in the control group of normal women. Citing the research of Morel, Magnan, and many others, Tarnovskaia also discussed the multitude of hereditary defects such as epilepsy, psychosis, idiocy, and others that indicated degeneration. However, of the 150 prostitutes interviewed for her study, 124 had alcoholic parents, making it the dominant hereditary factor.[32]

Tarnovskaia also examined the character of 100 of the 150 prostitutes in her study. From this examination she found that there was a weakening of intelligence and noticeable psychic abnormalities in most of these women. Most interesting were the few personal histories that were included in this study. As an example, Tarnovskaia told of Anna Z., whose father was an alcoholic and whose mother died of typhus when Anna was nine years old. At twelve, she was seduced by her employer at the laundry. Eventually, she became a maid for a midwife and took on a lover, but contracted urethritis and was abandoned by her lover at the hospital. Once Anna had recovered, she wanted to work at a brothel because a former classmate had told her that the life was easy. On her first attempt to enter a brothel, she was turned away because she was too young and the police returned her to the care of her father. Soon after, she left her father's house and found a brothel that would employ her. She eventually abandoned the brothel to follow a series of lovers. After these relationships ended, Anna again returned to the brothel. Tarnovskaia described Anna as having a face like a bird, with beautiful brown hair and sparkling, vivacious eyes.[33] Often these personal histories were accompanied by a photograph of the prostitute in question.

We might now read these case studies as part of the master narrative of degeneration that was particularly persuasive within Europe and Russia of the *fin de siècle*. Riccardo Nicolosi has posited that "case studies become indispensable elements of the explanation of the theory because they tell the *master narrative* [of degeneration] again and again and thereby 'confirm' it." The medical authority, in this case Tarnovskaia, provides a selective narrative that highlights specific events and pathological conditions in the life of the subject that simply corroborate the scientific theory of, in this case, criminality. Therefore, these narratives are telling not only of the lives of the patients (especially of women), but also how the phenomena of criminality were developed by medical authorities as a manifestation of degeneration.[34]

Part two of Tarnovskaia's study concentrated on female offenders who were interned in the Litovskii Zamok prison outside of St. Petersburg. As with the prostitutes, Tarnovskaia refused to accept that all criminals were the same, referencing the work of Lombroso, Orshanskii, and others, who wanted to distinguish the murderer from the forger. In this case, thieves were selected who had been repeat offenders. Tarnovskaia argued that the recurring nature of their crime once again suggested that they had not just stolen due to a singular incident or an unfortunate circumstance. Also, and more importantly, she felt that anatomically thieves shared a striking resemblance to prostitutes.

Once again, Tarnovskaia took issue with Lombroso's theory of the atavistic throwback, preferring the theories of Morel that suggested that degeneracy was a pathological phenomenon caused by the interaction of hereditary and environmental factors that were manifested in physical and mental deviations. According to Morel, families might display first neurasthenia or nervous hysteria, then alcohol and opiate addiction, leading to prostitution and criminal behavior, and finally resulting in insanity. Tarnovskaia preferred this approach to Lombroso's idea of arrested development as she desired to prove true deviations from the norm. Specifically, Morel offered hereditary defects as a possibility that would eliminate to some degree the influence of individual circumstance, national characteristics, social status, etc. With a special interest in heredity, Tarnovskaia argued that "the greater number of [her subjects] are part of a vast pathological family, which is subdivided into four morbid entities. Nervous and psychic patients. Prostitutes. Criminals. Alcoholics." What united these four groups of deviant women was a marked "psychic defectiveness" that was always accompanied by "physical and moral deviations" that distinguished them from normal women who were free of the hereditary taint of degeneration.[35]

As with the prostitutes, the thieves' personal histories contributed to the master narrative of degeneration. For example, Tarnovskaia provided the story of the thief Pauline who had "a rather pretty regular face although the expression is hard and nasty." Pauline was the daughter of an alcoholic laborer. Her mother had died when Pauline was seven years old. She was one of five children, four of whom had died in infancy. Two of the four died of scrofulous affections. Pauline grew up in squalor and often went hungry as her father remained a widower and drank away most of his pay. For a time, she was apprenticed to a seamstress and eventually learned her alphabet. At seventeen, however, she was accused of and sentenced for theft. She was imprisoned on a second offense when she stole a dozen handkerchiefs. She was arrested a third time for stealing clothes. Although she admitted to the thefts, Tarnovskaia noted that Pauline showed no remorse for her misdeeds or any comprehension of her culpability. This led Tarnovskaia to suggest that at twenty years old, Pauline was "a moral monster" who could commit crimes without flinching as long as the crime proved useful for her purposes. Pauline "is distinguished by a complete absence of benevolent ideas; [consumed] by excessive selfishness."[36]

In conclusion, Tarnovskaia pointed to environmental factors, specifically connecting them to the promiscuity, vice, and diseases of the parents, as well as to the complete lack of education for the children. Following from Morel, Tarnovskaia argued that heredity was an essential component—cruel and alcoholic parents were a particularly strong indicator of morally deviant children, especially if the mother was an alcoholic. Punishment of the offender was not enough, the environmental issues had to be addressed. Children must be taken away from the pernicious influence of cruel parents and the focus of philanthropic organizations should be on ridding a generation of the "morbid heredity" of moral and mental degeneration.[37] Interestingly, Tarnovskaia was advocating for social rejuvenation while supporting her conclusions with the objectivity of anthropometric methods. In this way, Tarnovskaia challenged Lombroso to think differently about social and biological factors.

From Lombroso, Tarnovskaia accepted the study of the born criminal. From Morel came consideration of hereditary factors associated with degeneration. Her focus on female offenders, however, was original and the argument for social reform that addressed public health issues was pioneering for the time. After all, Tarnovskaia was an important voice in the Russian scientific discourse that asserted that criminality could eventually be eradicated as a byproduct of an unhealthy social environment. Significantly, Nicolosi has argued that Russian criminal anthropologists tended to blend the theories of atavism and degeneration as complimentary, allowing for better narratives of criminality in their case studies.[38] Just as relevant, Beer has suggested that social reform and the transformation of members of society was so central to Russian progressive thought at this time that "[t]o condemn an entire criminal class of Russians to moral and social oblivion would have been an admission, at least in part, of the limited effects of social reform."[39] This is certainly the case in Taranovskaia's published research and, we might assume, in her conversations with Lombroso.

Soon after publication of *An Anthropological Study of Prostitutes and Female Thieves*, Tarnovskaia's work was positively reviewed in professional journals throughout the scientific world. In January 1891, the *Journal of Mental Science* published the following review, which I quote in full in order to reflect the way in which Tarnovskaia's research was received by her contemporaries:

> The author has recorded in this volume the results of his [*sic*] researches in the Hospital of Kalinkine and the Prison of Litowski Zamok. His [*sic*] observations extended over four years and were made on a great number of prostitutes and habitual female thieves. The methods of [Pierre Paul] Broca and [Paul] Topinard were adopted, and are set forth in great detail by means of drawings and comparative tables. The book constitutes another valuable contribution to the science of criminal anthropology and is the more valuable in that it consists mainly of definite ascertained facts.
>
> Dr Tarnowsky holds that it is necessary to know the origin and history of each individual case, and the stock from which she has sprung, before a conclusion of any value can be presented. He [*sic*] is of opinion that the parents, and even the forefathers, should have belonged not only to the same race, but also to the same country and province. The difficulties are still further augmented when it comes to be a question of the preponderance of morbid heredity, or the condition

of both the parents at the moment of conception, or of the psychical alterations that may exist in the person examined.

It is in fact, impossible to present the results of complete investigation. Impediments are inseparable from researches of this nature, and serious deficiencies in the chain of evidence must occur.

Dr Tarnowsky sets forth the reasons which have influenced him [*sic*] in his [*sic*] decision to study these persons in spite of the drawbacks above mentioned. These are briefly the uniformity of the race under observation, the anthropometric measurements, the anthropological characteristics, the hereditary influences, the extinction of the stock in the case of prostitutes as signs of degeneration, and the mental manifestations exhibited by these persons.

Prostitutes: Neater in personal appearance; comfort, good food, gew-gaws, pleasures and distractions are necessaries of life.
Work is abhorred by them; they live from hand to mouth.
They are expansive and sentimental.
General characteristics: laziness and absence of moral sense.

Thieves: Neither coquettes nor gourmands. They think little of comfort.
They work in prison and accumulate a little money against the day of their release.
They display energy and firmness, are more stable-minded, do not drink to such an excess as prostitutes.
A certain prudence, reserve, defiance, a want of sincerity, and absence of remorse are characteristic.
Denial of turpitude, and a certain amount of modesty is shown.

Dr Tarnowsky's observations on these two classes have been made on the same lines, and he [*sic*] arrives at the following conclusions:

1. Professional prostitutes are incomplete beings, having been arrested in development, tainted with a morbid heredity, and presenting signs of mental and bodily degeneration in connection with their imperfect evolution.
2. The signs of physical degeneration due to an imperfect organization are manifested by the frequency of malformation of the head, anomalies of the skull (41.33 per cent.), of the face (42.66 per cent.), of the ears (42 per cent.) and by defective teeth (54 per cent.).
3. Their mental anomalies are shown by more or less pronounced weakness of intellect, by a neurotic constitution, or by a notable absence of moral sense. These anomalies are confirmed by the abuse of the organs of generation, by the taste they show for their horrible business, to which they return voluntarily after having been set at liberty.
4. The signs of degeneration are more marked in the cases of those prostitutes and thieves whose mothers were habitual drunkards, and this confirms the theory that it is chiefly the influence of the mother that is re-echoed by the organism of the child.

5. The sterility and extinction of the stock of prostitutes depends in great measure on their abnormal condition—fertile in hereditary blemishes—which seems to confirm their degeneration.
6. Habitual prostitutes who cannot be classified with the sane and normal, since they make a business of such a life, fill up the two large gaps that criminal statistics establish in favour of women.
7. Habitual thieves, although also presenting a great number of the physical and moral signs which distinguish them from respectable women, nevertheless are not so far removed from the normal type as prostitutes. Because:
   a. The thieves are laden with a less pernicious heredity than the prostitutes.
   b. The signs of physical degeneration are fewer in number in thieves than in prostitutes
   c. The number of births is greater among the thieves.
   d. The principal diameters of the skull, as well as the total horizontal circumference, are greater amongst thieves than amongst prostitutes.
   e. The zygoma and jaw are larger among the prostitutes.
   f. The moral and intellectual level of thieves is higher than among the prostitutes. The thief has a greater self-respect—a more lively intelligence. She is more energetic, and brings a greater resistance into the struggle for life. She is much less lazy, and does not fear work
   g. However incorrigible the thief, however numerous her faults, she could not commit them and repeat them at all hours like the prostitute, it being granted that thieving and sexual vice are equal units—admitting for the moment that the two faults are of equal value. In every case the thief only steals at intervals, with the opportunity; while the prostitute traffics with her body without respite, and abandons the right to choose or to refuse—she does not wish to change her abject occupation.
8. Anthropometric results, as well as researches into their heredity, the circumstances of their birth, their subsequent social life, as well as the study of their intellectual and moral level, concur unanimously in proving that prostitutes and thieves belong to a class of women which is abnormal, degenerated, or degenerating. They are the products of the lower strata, of the refuse of society, and their number diminishes in proportion as evolution ameliorates mankind.

> The work of Dr Tarnowsky has cost him [*sic*] great labour and much time, and if it has not led to the results desiderated by the author, it nevertheless constitutes a highly meritorious production. It is apparent that these studies deserve every encouragement and are of great importance from a medicolegal point of view.[40]

The same year as this review, Tarnovskaia published in Russian *Thieves (An Anthropological Study)* (*Vorovki (antropologicheskoe issledovanie)*, 1891) and the following year *New Research on Criminal Anthropology* (*Novye raboty po kriminal'noi antropologii*, 1892).[41] It is doubtful that her American and European colleagues read these Russian works.

Nevertheless, French criminologists who had criticized Lombroso's theory of the born criminal could not ignore Tarnovskaia's detailed research that blended atavism with degeneration. Soon, French researchers were making similar connections between the prostitute and the criminal. More specifically, Octave Simonot extended the theory of the born prostitute using Tarnovskaia's anthropometric approach in his study "The Physiological Psychology of Prostitution" (Psychologie physiologique de la prostitueé, 1911). Simonot focused his research on disturbances in cerebral activity and argued that just as among savages, prostitutes survived on "spontaneous attention" which could be linked to distraction and susceptibility to idées fixes, clear symptoms of degeneracy. As Alain Corbin has noted, Tarnovskaia, Simonot, and others accepted the primacy of the biological with environmental factors contributing to a hereditary inevitability. Essentially, prostitution was an inherited predisposition.[42] In fact, Tarnovskaia would explicitly posit this argument in a later work, *Women Who Kill* (*Zhenshchiny-ubiitsy*), that atavism might be a predisposition for criminality, rather than a biological *fait accompli*.

In November 1891, Tarnovskaia sent a letter from St. Petersburg to Lombroso stating that she had the photographs and anthropometric measurements of criminal women needed for an article that was to appear in his journal *The Archive of Psychiatry, Criminal Sciences and Criminal Anthropology* (*Archivio di psichiatria, scienze penali ed antropologia criminale*). As part of this research effort, Tarnovskaia expressed her gratitude for being given the opportunity to collaborate with other criminal anthropologists.[43] In fact, Lombroso and Salvatore Ottolenghi (1861–1934) would publish *The Criminal Woman and the Prostitute* (*La donna delinquente e la prostituta*), in which some of the data (measurements and anomalies of female criminals) was provided by Tarnovskaia. Over the next two years, Tarnovskaia, Lombroso, and Ottolenghi would (independently and jointly) publish in *The Archive of Psychiatry* several works on female offenders (more on this below).

During the writing of *Criminal Woman*, Lombroso wrote to Tarnovskaia and expressed his gratitude for the data that she had sent to him. He claimed that he could not have written his book had it not been for her help. Lombroso also wrote that he would not attend the third *International Congress of Criminal Anthropology* in Brussels (1892). With a backhanded compliment, Lombroso stated that Tarnovskaia was one of the rare exceptions to the inferiority of women with respect to men. In fact, Lombroso seemed to acknowledge the

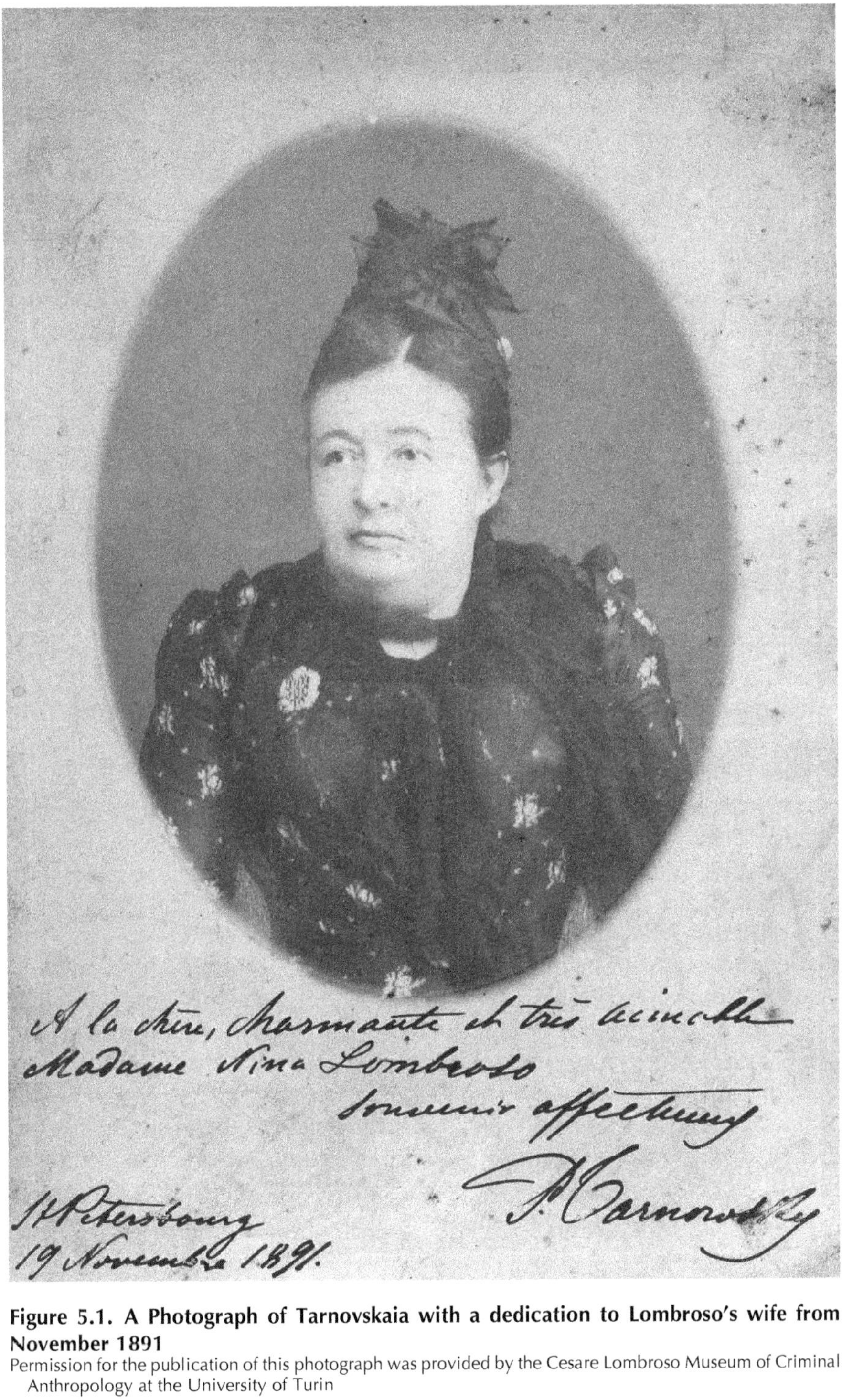
A la chère, charmante et très aimable
Madame Nina Lombroso
souvenir affectueux
P. Tarnowsky
St Petersbourg
19 Novembre 1891.

Figure 5.1. A Photograph of Tarnovskaia with a dedication to Lombroso's wife from November 1891
Permission for the publication of this photograph was provided by the Cesare Lombroso Museum of Criminal Anthropology at the University of Turin

"genius" of Tarnovskaia's research, even stating that the doctors (mainly men) attending the Brussels conference only knew half as much as Tarnovskaia on the subject of criminality.[44]

The French contingent's challenge at the second congress contributed to the absence of the Italian scholars at the congress in Brussels. At the third congress, several reports argued against Lombroso's born criminal type, suggesting that dividing individuals into criminals and non-criminals was arbitrary. Although some criminals did present pathological and degenerative characteristics, they did not constitute a special category of degenerates. As a result, Lombroso would be forced to defend (or to further develop) both his theory of the born criminal and his classification of the criminal type.[45]

Although Lombroso did not attend the *International Congress of Criminal Anthropology*, Tarnovskaia did, where she presented the paper "On the Sense Organs of Criminal Women" (Sur les organes des sens chez les femmes criminelles). Tarnovskaia investigated vision, taste, sense of smell, hearing, tactile and pain sensitivity in female murderers and prostitutes. Her findings were inconclusive and most of the respondents at the conference believed that there was no discernable difference in the sensitivity found in criminals and non-criminals. Tarnovskaia, however, was congratulated by her colleagues for taking these sensory measurements as a new frontier for future scholarly research. Her paper and the following discussion were published in French as part of the conference proceedings.[46]

After the conference, on November 23, 1892, Tarnovskaia sent a copy of her presentation to Lombroso to be published in *The Archive of Psychiatry*, although it never appeared, possibly because the findings were not conclusive. Writing from St. Petersburg, Tarnovskaia also asked if the photographs that she had sent had arrived.[47] In 1893, Tarnovskaia's "The Physiognomy of the Russian Prostitute" (Fisionomie di prostitute russe) and a co-authored piece with Lombroso (with the just mentioned photographs), "Photographs of Russian Criminals" (Fotografie di criminali russe), were published in Italian in *The Archive of Psychiatry*. Both of these articles had direct relevance for Lombroso and Ferrero's project on female offenders.

In 1893, *Criminal Woman* was published in Italian with a Russian translation available two years later.[48] In this influential work, Lombroso and Ferrero attempted to identify the female criminal type. According to this research, only 18 percent of female criminals displayed the stigmata of degeneration (making them born criminals), but when prostitutes were added, the number increased to 37 percent. Lombroso and Ferrero argued that the female born criminal was more savage than the male born criminal, characterizing these women as vengeful and cruel. As Horn has noted, Lombroso asserted that he could identify dangerous women with scientific comparisons to criminal men, children, "savages," and nonhuman primates. However, rather than providing a transparent pathology of the female criminal, Lombroso and Ferrero provided "the barely legible *potential* dangerousness of the normal woman."[49]

Significant for this chapter, Lombroso was deeply indebted to the earlier research and efforts of "Pauline Tarnowsky," which is evident throughout *Criminal Woman.* Possibly of greatest importance were the photographs of prostitutes provided by Tarnovskaia as Italy prohibited the measuring, photographing, or studying of criminals once they had been convicted.[50] Using the photographs, Lombroso and Ferrero noted that the Russian prostitutes were more beautiful than the female criminals. The scarcity of the criminal type among the prostitutes was explained by the fact that prostitutes had to be appealing to male clients. Also, prostitutes knew how to use make-up and their youth to minimize degenerative characteristics. However, the authors of this study warned, "[w]hen youth vanishes, those jaws, those cheekbones and sharp angles hidden by adipose tissues emerge and the face becomes virile, uglier than that of a man. Then the wrinkles deepen, becoming like scars, and the once pleasant face fully reveals the degenerative type into which it was born."[51]

Just as important were the anthropometric measurements that seemed to indicate criminality. In chapter 14, *Anthropometry of Female Criminals*, and chapter 15, *Facial and Cephalic Anomalies of Female Criminals and Prostitutes*, Lombroso and Ferrero referred directly to Tarnovskaia's published research of 1889 as a basis for their own findings. They also acknowledged the collaborative research project with Tarnovskaia that had involved 69 female criminals and 100 Moscow prostitutes that had informed Lombroso and Ottolenghi's *The Criminal Woman and the Prostitute*.[52] In chapter 14, Lombroso and Ferrero asserted that Tarnovskaia's research "confirms the prevalence of small cranial capacities among prostitutes" with reference to her measurements of thieves, prostitutes, illiterate peasants, and 50 educated moral women. As well, Tarnovskaia's research showed that there were more blond prostitutes than thieves, because fair-haired prostitutes were more sought after.[53]

In chapter 16, *Other Anomalies*, Lombroso and Ferrero deferred to Tarnovskaia's finding on the cleft palate as a significant characteristic of degeneration. Similarly, asymmetrical eyebrows were noted by Tarnovskaia in 44 percent of prostitutes, 40 percent of suicides, 20 percent of thieves, and 4 percent of normal women.[54] In chapter 18, *The Criminal Type in Women and Its Atavistic Origins*, Lombroso and Ferrero again turned to the research findings of Tarnovskaia, referencing the measurements of the 150 St. Petersburg prostitutes and the 100 Moscow prostitutes, which they combined with the work of other anthropologists in order to ascertain the frequency of these atavistic markers. As noted above, by adding prostitutes to their taxonomy, the stigmata of degeneration rose to 37 percent of those women under consideration. Horn has argued that the prostitute was added by Lombroso and Ferrero as the true expression of female degeneration in order to overcome two apparent contradictions: proportionally, there were too few female criminals and these female criminals rarely displayed anatomical signs of social deviance.[55]

It is more likely that the two Italians were repeating the distinctions offered by Tarnovskaia, who along with her husband specialized in Russian prostitution. It must be remembered that Tarnovskaia's initial interest was in the registered prostitute who chose this profession (a born prostitute) even after being given an opportunity to change her circumstances. The original goal was to find the mental or physical defect through anthropometric measurements and hereditary factors. Tarnovskaia had written in 1889: "By plying their trade, inveterate prostitutes, whom one cannot consider healthy, normal, or honest, fill the excessively large gap that criminal statistics create in favor of women. We believe that inveterate prostitutes supply the counterweight that balances the criminal scales and distributes crime more evenly and fairly between the two sexes."[56] Frankly, it was Tarnovskaia and other European criminologists who had introduced prostitutes to the scientific discourse of "criminals" prior to the publication of *Criminal Woman*—not just a way in which Lombroso and Ferrero could inflate the number of female offenders.[57]

In chapter 20, Lombroso and Ferrero privileged Tarnovskaia's data on menstruation (because she was a woman and collected the data herself), in which it was confirmed that "prostitutes menstruate prematurely." The two male authors of *Criminal Woman* asserted that "[m]enstruation strongly influences certain crimes."[58] Similarly, Tarnovskaia's research contributed to measures such as the sensitivity to pain,[59] hearing,[60] dress,[61] occasional crime,[62] moral insanity, and hysteria among prostitutes.[63]

Beyond Tarnovskaia's influence noted above, we also know that Lombroso believed that there were affinities between Russia and the newly established Kingdom of Italy. Lombroso believed that the large rural population in both countries fostered more brutal crime and vigilantism.[64] In fact, Pick argues that much of Lombroso's research was influenced by the social issues acknowledged during Italian unification; a mainly illiterate peasant population was ruled by a class that was linguistically isolated from them. For Lombroso, national unity would be achieved by distinguishing those who could not become part of the new Italy.[65] A similar socio-political situation between an illiterate peasantry and a Europeanized aristocracy was occurring in Russia. Marina Mogilner notes that Tarnovskaia's research acknowledged a prejudice for purely racially Russian subjects. At the same time, her colleagues and fellow followers of Lombroso such as Kovalevskii, Chizh, and Ivan Sikorskii

(1845–1919) were championing a type of Russian biological nationalism.[66] Therefore, Lombroso might have more readily accepted the data and findings of Tarnovskaia given these perceived socio-political similarities.

Pick states that Lombroso's willingness to accept elements of the French theory of degeneration that stressed environmental corruption reflected a growing disenchantment with the efforts made toward a unified Italy. As social problems were magnified with the rapid expansion of cities, atavism seemed to address localized problems of banditry, provincialism, and superstition. Nevertheless, Lombroso did not revise his earlier work, but incorporated the research on degeneration into later editions of *Criminal Man* even while his central thesis remained intact.[67]

The affinity with Russia might have been further strengthened by Lombroso's conversations with family friend Anna Kulisheva (1857–1925; Kuliscioff), a leading feminist and militant Marxist. Notably, Lombroso referenced Kulisheva's lecture "The Monopoly of Men" in *Criminal Woman*. The lecture took issue with measuring intelligence by measuring the size of the brain. Kulisheva, like Tarnovskaia, believed that environmental and social factors, like the lack of educational opportunities for women, more significantly contributed to the supposed lower intelligence of women.[68]

Arguably, Lombroso willingly embraced Tarnovskaia's research, which along with the French criticism encouraged him to change some of his original scientific assertions on atavism. It seems certain that Lombroso, under the influence of Tarnovskaia's *An Anthropological Study of Prostitutes and Female Thieves*, not only applied his theory of the born criminal to women, but also included photographs to demonstrate the physical anomalies, introduced a control group of normal women, and reached many of the very same conclusions as his Russian colleague.

At the 1896 *International Congress of Criminal Anthropology* held in Geneva, Tarnovskaia presented a paper on female criminality that invited a discussion with the leading figures of the field including Lombroso himself. From the published version of this presentation, it appears that Tarnovskaia did not include prostitutes in her presentation. Instead, this presentation referred only to female murderers and anticipated *Women Who Kill*, which was to be published six years later. Even at this point of a new project, Tarnovskaia understood that social conditions and a lack of educational opportunities for women were significant factors in any discussion of female criminality. For example, Tarnovskaia noted that mariticide (killing of one's husband) was very common in rural Russia due to the forced marriages of very young peasant girls by their parents. She noted that under the law, the male and female murderer of a spouse were treated the same. However, the husband maintained a superior position within the home (outside of the law)

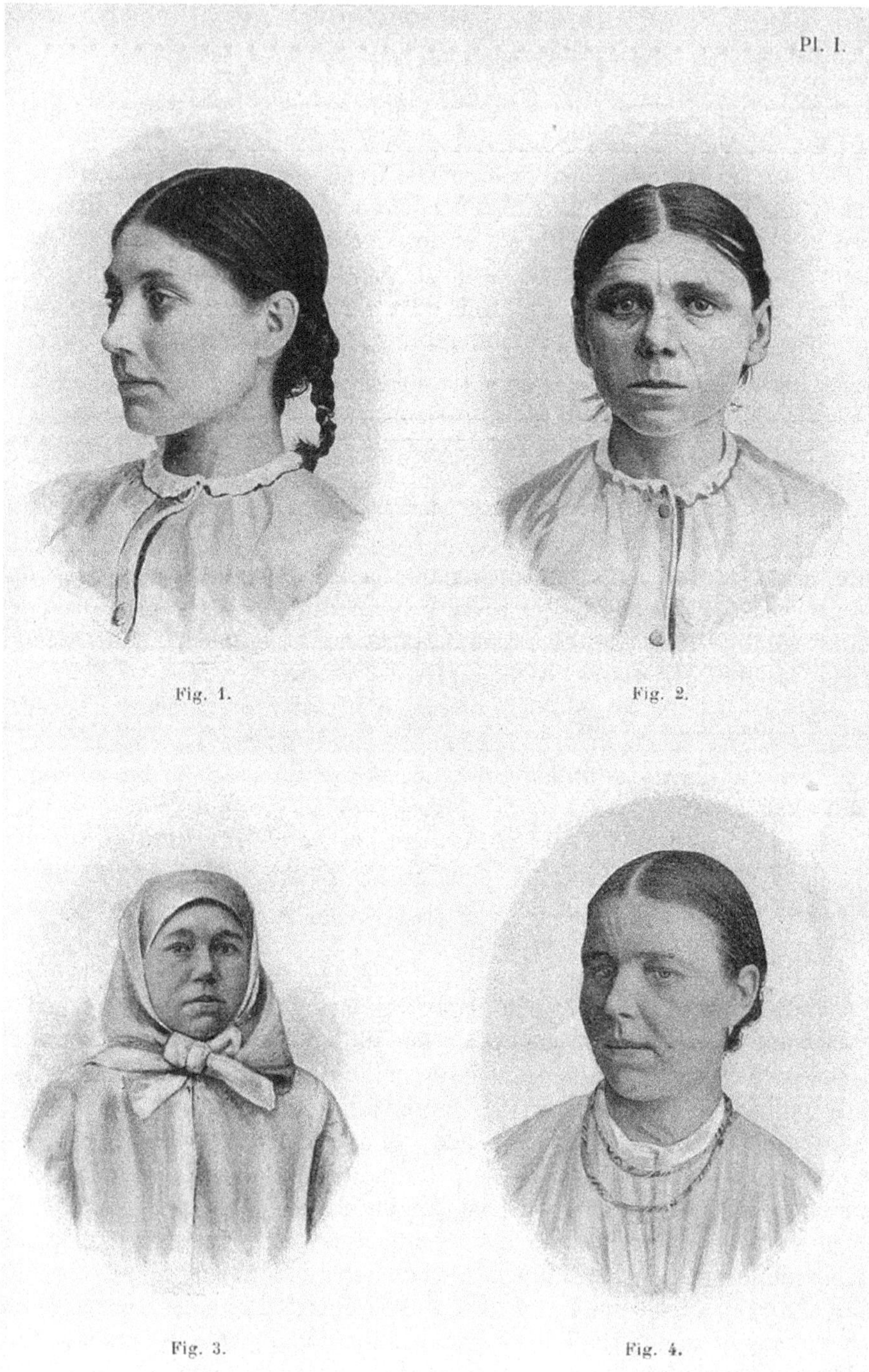

Figure 5.2. Russian female murderers depicted in Tarnovskaia's *Women Who Kill*
Etude anthropométrique sur les Prostituées et les Voleuses, 1889

and as divorce was not allowed for the rural population, mariticide occurred at a significantly higher rate than uxoricide (the killing of one's wife).

Tarnovskaia spent the final part of her presentation defending criminal anthropology from critics whom she said was asking too much of a new science. Criminal anthropology must be allowed to evolve and to develop as had other sciences. Having made her presentation, Lombroso asked Tarnovskaia several questions about male and female crime. Tarnovskaia stated that for domestic and petty crime there was no significant difference in rates between men and women. Men were more often involved in "accidental" crimes due to their greater physical strength and the frequent occurrence of alcohol, while women tended to be involved in more premediated crimes, mainly because of their lower position in society.[69]

The following year, Lombroso came to Moscow for the *International Medical Congress.* Most attention has been paid to this visit by those interested in the meeting of Lombroso with the writer Lev Tolstoy at his estate in the Tula region.[70] Less has been said about his meeting with Russian criminal anthropologists. For several days, however, Lombroso remained in Moscow and met with his Russian colleagues. More than likely, Tarnovskaia came down from St. Petersburg for the conference or, at least, to visit with Lombroso. At forty-eight, Tarnovskaia was a well-known and respected physician and researcher, who had contributed greatly to the popularization of Lombroso's theories in Russia and in Europe.

In 1902, Tarnovskaia published *Women Who Kill* in Russian, in which she argued that predicting criminality was multifactorial. In so doing, she rejected Lombroso's original assertion of a born criminal type as the lone determining factor. Tarnovskaia acknowledged that there were social factors (lack of education and deplorable living conditions), anatomical data, moral deviations, heredity, and much more that contributed to criminal behavior. She suggested, however, that criminal anthropology played a role in identifying an individual's *predisposition* for criminality. If one were to reframe the discussion in these terms, then there was a place for Lombroso's typology of the criminal.[71]

As in her earlier research, Tarnovskaia wished to emphasize the distinction between criminal activity caused by circumstance and the recidivism of the career criminal. However, she also acknowledged that the science of criminal anthropology was still in its infancy and that more study was necessary to be able to react properly to those predisposed to crime. One of the confounding factors was the demand of the legal system to provide definitive answers, sometimes well before the scientific community had reached agreement. Tarnovskaia understood that her research and the research of others was only part of the development of criminal anthropology as a science and acknowledged that her work was part of the "material" that still awaited a "future architect" who would synthesize the various materials into a coherent structure.[72]

Later in her study, Tarnovskaia organized the achievements of Lombroso and his school of researchers in similar terms. Lombroso had successfully gathered theories and data from various strains of scientific research and, maybe more importantly, had presented his ideas about criminality in ways that were meaningful for both the legal and medical communities. Significantly, Tarnovskaia argued one could choose to agree or disagree with his ideas, but no one could ignore Lombroso. This was a significant statement considering that Tarnovskaia, herself, may well have been much more innovative and rigorous in her research methods, but possibly lacked the ability to catch "the attention of doctors and lawyers on the issue of the psychic imbalance of criminals."[73] Clearly, Tarnovskaia understood Lombroso as the master architect, who had used her research (materials) and that of others to build the grand structure that was the new science of criminal anthropology.

Even as "an innovator of great talent," Lombroso had critics who stubbornly attacked his ideas, but he also had "hard-working students and colleagues working to expand the new scientific branch, which he has created."[74] Tarnovskaia then provided a summary of the various important moments in the development of criminal anthropology with reference to the congresses in Paris, Brussels, Rome, and Geneva, where Lombroso's opponents attacked aspects of his scientific theory. Taking the main critics individually, mainly from the French school, Tarnovskaia defended Lombroso and articulated how his theories evolved over time. Just as important, she presented a compelling argument as to how science would change legal definitions of crime, the organization of judicial categories, and the sentencing of criminals.

Beer has suggested that Russian practitioners of the human sciences were frustrated by the lack of funding, the political interference, and the failure of the tsarist bureaucracy to implement changes to the criminal codes and to reform medical and psychiatric care. As a result, the intersecting disciplines of anthropology, psychiatry, psychology, criminology, jurisprudence, and sociology directed their energies to examine the spread of crime and subversion that hindered the maturation of Russian society. The existence of a large population of degenerate individuals in society, so the argument went, limited the opportunities for liberal reform. "Accordingly, the human sciences came to articulate strategies for the attainment of national emancipation and harmony, predicated on the gradual transformation not simply of the empire's social, economic, and political structures but, ultimately, of its human population as well."[75] This belief was clearly evident in Tarnovskaia's argument that criminal anthropology might inform the development of better legal, penal, and medical systems within the larger context of social reform.

Tarnovskaia's work was published in French translation in 1908, making it more accessible to American and European scientists. The study involved 160 females involved in murder and included anthropometric measurements, sensory tests (sight, hearing, smell, taste, general and pain sensitivity, spacial orientation, reflexes, and muscular strength), and personal histories. There was also a control group of peasant women selected from central Russia. Tarnovskaia also noted the stigmata of degeneration, both the physical and the moral markers as originally identified by Morel. She concentrated on crimes that were mainly associated with female offenders—murder of the husband (often precipitated by reproductive or sexual issues) and infanticide. She concluded that among the majority of the females who committed murder there were hereditary factors and a congenital predisposition for crime (expressed in various forms of psychic imbalance).

Tarnovskaia organized female crime within her study into four main categories: Crimes of passion with seven subcategories (involving greed, maternal love, sexual love, jealousy, vengeance, repeated insults or hatred, and cruelty); altered perception with two subcategories (atrophy of morals and genetic deviations); accidental killings; and nervous and psychiatric disorders.[76] Once again, contemporary readers might be less interested in anthropometric data and a discussion of early or late menstruation among criminal women, but the personal histories offer remarkable medical narratives for these women at the beginning of the twentieth century.

For example, observation XV: Anna Vasil'eva Neugoda was 35 years old and sentenced to four years of hard labor for the attempted murder of the peasant Alexander Petrov. Heredity: Neugoda did not know her father, who died before she was born. Her mother had recently died of typhoid fever. The couple had four children, two of whom died at a young age. Personal history: Neugoda was illiterate. She had married twice, the first time at nineteen. The sudden death of her first husband was noticed in the village and some believed that she had poisoned him. Neugoda remarried and had four children, two of whom remained living. She denied taking part in the attempted murder of Alexander Petrov and considered herself wrongly convicted. However, the peasant Petrov ate a cranberry cake, made by his wife, and soon after was sick and vomiting. Suspecting his wife of poisoning him, the peasant questioned her and learned that she had bought arsenic from Neugoda for a ruble. Supposedly, Neugoda had stated to Petrov's wife that it was with arsenic that she had killed her first husband. Arsenic was found upon examining the cake that had been given to Petrov. When Neugoda's house was searched, various herbs and pharmaceutical drugs were found. Neugoda was accused of collusion in the attempted murder of Petrov. Neugoda was found guilty but maintained her innocence.

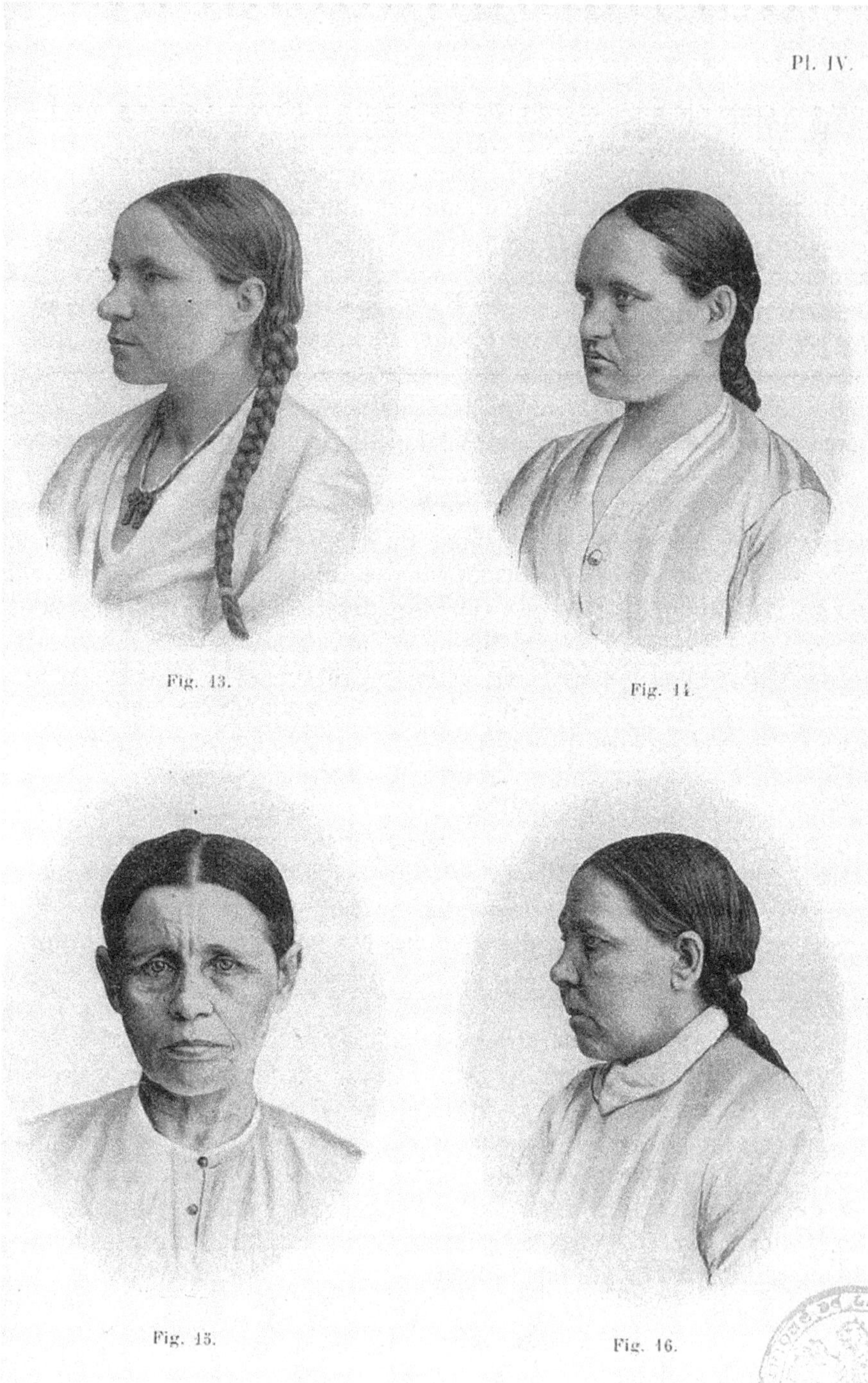

Figure 5.3. Anna Vasil'eva Neugoda
Etude anthropométrique sur les Prostituées et les Voleuses, 1889

In her conclusion of *Women Who Kill*, Tarnovskaia again addressed specific critics of criminal anthropology and admitted some mistakes that had been made in earlier research. For example, she acknowledged that it was necessary to add a control group to such studies. She reiterated that heredity factors and a psychic imbalance were evident in almost all of the women, but she also noted that sociological factors most likely were strong contributors like the forced marriages of young girls, the prevalence of sexual assault by the father-in-law in peasant communities, the beatings of young girls by mothers- and fathers-in-law, and more such indignities. These were so severe that some women might believe that a significant prison sentence was easier to accept. Tarnovskaia believed that in time, with further development of the methodology, criminal anthropology might inform the court system, penal reform, and medical treatment. With refinement of the scientific methodology, it would become easy to identify and categorize various groups of criminals and degenerates on a large scale.

Soon after its publication in French, *Women Who Kill* was positively reviewed by American and European colleagues. Adolph Meyer (1866–1950), who was the director of the Pathological Institute of the New York State Hospital system, said of Tarnovskaia's book: "From a methodological viewpoint and as a substantial contribution of facts, the volume is a great help for concrete orientation in this field."[77] Meyer would become the first psychiatrist-in-chief at Johns Hopkins Hospital in 1910. The criminologist Charles Goring (1870–1919) credited Tarnovskaia for her "conscientious industry, which insures reliability, [. . .] combined with the excellent arrangement and lucid exposition of her facts." Despite noting Tarnovskaia's significant "spade-work," Goring took issue with "the spirit of partisanship of the old school of criminologists," by which he meant Lombroso and his followers, found in Tarnovskaia's book.[78] A few years later, Goring would publish *The English Convict: A Statistical Study* (1913), which refuted Lombroso's assertions, arguing that there was no such thing as an anthropological criminal type.[79] Arthur MacDonald (1856–1936), an ardent supporter of Lombroso, provided a brief summary of Tarnovskaia's book and called her "the only woman criminologist of the world."[80] MacDonald was the author of *Criminology* (1892), the first American book that examined the causation of criminality.[81]

Clearly, Tarnovskaia's scholarly works were read and reviewed by the leading researchers of the time. She was recognized as one of the foremost experts within the field and even if some, like Goring, did not support the theories of the born criminal, no one seemed to refute the data that Tarnovskaia had collected, data that informed her opinions. The same year that MacDonald published his review, Tarnovskaia passed away in St. Petersburg.

In an obituary that was published in the *Journal of the American Institute of Criminal Law and Criminology*, she was called "the leading woman criminologist of Europe." It was also noted that she was an active and influential participant at international congresses and a frequent collaborator with Lombroso, Enrico Ferri (1856–1929), and other Italian criminologists.[82]

In conclusion, Tarnovskaia's research had a significant influence on Lombroso and his theories on female criminals. Even if Tarnovskaia saw Lombroso as the master architect who had successfully gained the attention of the legal and medical professions, it was her meticulous "spade-work" (as Goring called it) and willingness to respond to scholarly criticism in order to evolve the methods and theories of criminal anthropology that informed the greater discussion of female prostitutes, thieves, and murderers. In so doing, Tarnovskaia was recognized in the West as a leading criminal anthropologist, whose work was appreciated even by those who were skeptical of Lombroso's theory of atavism. Finally, Tarnovskaia's research is still interesting today if we concentrate on the personal histories of the hundreds of Russian women who were measured, photographed, and interviewed for these studies. In these narratives and in Tarnovskaia's own research, we recognize the deleterious impacts of alcoholism and poor healthcare and the lack of educational opportunities among the poor and especially among poor women. We can appreciate that prostitution, theft, and even murder might have been the only option that many of these women felt that they had in a society that offered few legitimate prospects for a successful and fulfilling life. We might also re-read many of these personal histories as part of what Nicolosi calls the master narrative of degeneration.[83] As a result, we should appreciate the significant contribution that Tarnovskaia made to science and the study of women and acknowledge the substantial role that she played in the evolution of Lombroso's own research on criminality.

NOTES

1. Kowalsky, Sharon A., *Deviant Women,* Dekalb: Northern University Press, 2009, 40–47.

2. In fact, not much has been written about Tarnovskaia. In the extant scholarship on Lombroso, it is often noted that Tarnovskaia and her scholarly influence warrant more research. In scholarship on Russian criminology, Tarnovskaia gets little more than a passing mention. In these publications, Tarnovskaia is discussed in some detail: Bernstein, Laurie, *Sonia's Daughters: Prostitutes and Their Regulation in Imperial Russia,* Berkeley: University of California Press, 1995, 126–128; Engelstein, Laura, *The Keys to Happiness. Sex and the Search for Modernity in Fin-de-Siècle Russia,* Ithaca, 1992, 133–154; Gilman, Sander L., *Difference and Pathology: Stereotypes of*

Sexuality, Race and Madness, Ithaca: Cornell University Press, 1985, 94–101; Mogilner, Marina, *Homo Imperii: A History of Physical Anthropology in Russia,* Lincoln: University of Nebraska Press, 2013, 339–341; Rafter, Nicole, ed., *The Origins of Criminology: A Reader,* New York: Routledge, 2009, 178–181.

3. I would like to express my deep appreciation to Silvano Montaldo, Professor of History and Director of the Lombroso Museum in Turino. Professor Montaldo provided valuable materials and insights for this chapter.

4. Beer, Daniel, "Blueprints for Change: The Human Sciences and the Coercive Transformation of Deviants in Russia, 1890–1930," *Osiris*, vol. 22, no. 1 (2007): 26–47; 30–31.

5. Hatchen, Elizabeth A., "In Service to Science and Society: Scientists and the Public in Late-Nineteenth-Century Russia," *Osiris*, 2nd Series, vol. 17, Science and Civil Society (2002): 171–209.

6. Beer, Daniel, *Renovating Russia: The Human Sciences and the Fate of Liberal Modernity 1880–1930*, Ithaca: Cornell University Press, 2008, 33.

7. Horn, David G., *The Criminal Body: Lombroso and the Anatomy of Deviance,* New York: Routledge, 2003, 5.

8. Biographical information on Orshanskii can be found on many websites including the online Russian biographical encyclopedia. See *Biografiia.ru: naibolee polnoe sobraniie biografii*, http://www.biografija.ru/show_bio.aspx?id=101640. Last accessed on July 2, 2018.

9. Sirotkina, Irina, *Diagnosing Literary Genius. A Cultural History of Psychiatry in Russia, 1880–1930*, Baltimore: The Johns Hopkins University Press, 2002, 61; 65.

10. Iudin, T., *Ocherki istorii otechestvennoi psikhiatrii*, Moscow: Medgiz, 1951, 138.

11. Kowalsky, *Deviant Women*, 207–208.

12. Bogdanov, Konstantin, *Vrachi, patsienty, chitateli: Patograficheskie teksty russkoi kul'tury XVIII–XIX vekov,* Moscow: O.G.I., 2005, 262–263; Sirotkina, *Diagnosing Literary Genius*, 23–35; 57–65; 79–82; Beer, Daniel, "The Medicalization of Religious Deviance in the Russian Orthodox Church (1880–1905)," *Kritika: Explorations in Russian and Eurasian History*, vol. 5, no. 3 (Summer 2004): 451–482, 468.

13. Mogilner, *Homo Imperii,* 241–245.

14. Dril', Dmitrii, *Maloletnye prestupniki, Etiud po voprosu o chelovecheskoi prestupnosti, ee fektorakh, i sredstvakh bor'by s nei,* 2 vols., Moscow: Tip. A. I. Mamontova i Ko., 1884–1888; *Prestupnost' i prestupniki (Ugolovno-psikhologicheskie etiudy),* St. Petersburg: Izdanie Ia. Kantorovicha, 1895.

15. Sirotkina, *Diagnosing Literary Genius*, 23–24.

16. Engelstein, *The Keys to Happiness,* 133–154; Rafter, *The Origins of Criminology,* 178–181.

17. Kowalsky, *Deviant Women*, 28.

18. Beer, "Blueprints for Change," 33.

19. Lombroso, Cesare and Gulielmo Ferrero, *Criminal Woman, the Prostitute and the Normal Woman*, translated and introduced by Nicole Hahn Rafter and Mary Gibson, Durham: Duke University Press, 2004, 23. Also see Wolfgang, Marvin E,. "Pioneers in Criminology: Cesare Lombroso (1835–1909)," *The Journal of Criminal*

Law, Criminology, and Police Science, vol. 52, no. 4 (November–December 1961): 361–391, 381; Lindsey, Edward, "The International Congress of Criminal Anthropology: A Review," *Journal of the American Institute of Criminal Law and Criminology,* vol. 1, no. 4 (November 1910): 578–583, 578–579.

20. Pick, Daniel, *Faces of Degeneration: A European Disorder, c. 1848–c. 1918,* Cambridge: Cambridge University Press, 1989, 112–113; 132–133; 136–137.

21. Sirotkina, *Diagnosing Literary Genius*, 23–25.

22. Bialkowski, Zygmunt Ronald, "The Transformation of Academic Criminal Jurisprudence into Criminology in Late Imperial Russia," PhD Dissertation, University of California, Berkeley, Fall 2007, 86.

23. Tarnovskaia, P.N. [Tarnowsky, Pauline], *Étude anthropométrique sur les prostituées et les voleuses*, Paris: Progrés Mèdical, 1889. Tarnovskaia had published this research the previous year in Russian: Tarnovskaia, P.N., "Antropometricheskie issledovaniia prostitutok, vorovok i zdorovykh krest'ianok-polevykh rabotnits (zasedanie 21 noiabria 1887 g.)," in *Protokoly zasedanii obshchestva psikhiatrov v S.-Peterburge za 1887 god,* St. Petersburg, 1888.

24. Gilman, *Difference and Pathology,* 94–101; quote: 98.

25. Marina Mogilner argues that in this designation of normative and deviant groups, Tarnovskaia used ethnicity as an organizing factor thereby adding a political implication to the notion of a Russian "born criminal." This approach was not limited to Tarnovskaia and, as Mogilner argues, became a way for authorities to reorganize and to control Imperial diversity. See both Mogilner, *Homo Imperii,* 339–341; Mogilner, Marina, "The Empire-Born Criminal. Atavism, Survivals, Irrational Instincts, and the Fate of Russian Imperial Modernity," in *Born to be Criminal,* edited by Nicolosi and Hartmann, 31–62, 36–37.

26. Marvin E. Wolfgang has argued that in the first edition of *Criminal Man,* Lombroso relied solely on anatomical and anthropometric data with a focus on the theory of atavism. However, in later editions, Lombroso adopted concepts of degeneration as one of the causes of criminality. Wolfgang, "Pioneers in Criminology," 374.

27. Tarnovskaia [Tarnowsky], *Étude anthropométrique sur les prostituées et les voleuses*, 9.

28. It is important to note the establishment of the school of moral statistics by Adolphe Quetelet (1796–1874) and André-Michel Guerry (1802–1866), who had been using national crime statistics provided by the French government. Rates of crime in France had varied little from year to year, leading Quetelet and Guerry to assert that biological and social factors might be the cause of crime. Interestingly, Wolfgang argues that there is no convincing evidence that Lombroso influenced Quetelet and Guerry or vice versa. Wolfgang, "Pioneers in Criminology," 368.

29. Mogilner, *Homo Imperii*, 328–331; Mailis, N.P., *Osnovy daktiloskopii. Kurs lektsii,* Moscow: RGUP, 2016, 16–17.

30. Tarnovskaia [Tarnowsky], *Étude anthropométrique sur les prostituées et les voleuses*, 23.

31. Ibid., 26.

32. Ibid., 49.

33. Ibid., 76–77.

34. Nicolosi, Riccardo, "Criminality, Deviance, and Anthropological Diversity: Narratives of Inborn Criminality and Atavism in Late Imperial Russia (1880–1900)," in *Born to be Criminal,* edited by Nicolosi and Hartmann, 85–116, 92.

35. Tarnovskaia [Tarnowsky], *Étude anthropométrique sur les prostituées et les voleuses*, 107–108.

36. Ibid., 120.

37. Ibid., 195; 197; 204.

38. Nicolosi, "Criminality, Deviance, and Anthropological Diversity," 93.

39. Beer, "Blueprints for Change," 34.

40. "'Étude anthropométrique sur les prostituées et les voleuses.' By Dr Pauline Tarnowsky. Progrés Mèdical 1889," *The Journal of Mental Science*, no. 157, vol. XXXVII (April 1891): 265–268. Also see a review of Tarnovskaia's book in *The American Journal of Insanity*, vol. 47, no. I–F (1890): 82.

41. Tarnovskaia, P.N., *Vorovki (antropologicheskoe issledovanie),* St. Petersburg: Tipografiia doma prezreniia maloletnikh bednykh, 1891.

42. Corbin, Alain, *Women for Hire. Prostitution and Sexuality in France after 1850,* translated by Alan Sheridan, Cambridge: Harvard University Press, 1990, 304–308.

43. The letter is part of the #Lombroso Project, IT SMAUT Ferrero/CL. 98, http://www.lombrosoproject.unito.it/eng/dtl.php?id=4336; The original is held by Museo di antropologia criminale "Cesare Lombroso"—Università di Torino.

44. The letter is part of the #Lombroso Project, IT SMAUT Carrara/CL.—Lombroso, Cesare 46, http://www.lombrosoproject.unito.it/eng/dtl.php?id=5470; The original is held by Museo di antropologia criminale "Cesare Lombroso"—Università di Torino.

45. Lindsey, "The International Congress of Criminal Anthropology," 579–580.

46. Tarnovskaia, P.N., "Sur les organes des sens chez les femmes criminelles," in *Actes du troisième congrès international d'anthropologie criminelle tenu a Bruxellesen aout 1892*. Brussels: F. Hayez, 1893: 224–233, 233–235.

47. The letter is part of the #Lombroso Project, IT SMAUT Carrara/CL.—Tarnowsky, Pauline 01, http://www.lombrosoproject.unito.it/eng/dtl.php?id=5648; The original is held by Museo di antropologia criminale "Cesare Lombroso"—Università di Torino.

48. Lombroso, Cesare and Gulielmo Ferrero, *Zhenshchina prestupnitsa i prostitutka,* translated and introduced by Dr. G.I. Gordon, Kiev; Kharkov: F.I. Ioganson, 1897.

49. Horn, David G., "This Norm Is Not One: Reading the Female Body in Lombroso's Anthropology," in *Deviant Bodies: Critical Perspectives on Difference in Science and Popular Culture,* edited by Jennifer Terry and Jacqueline Urla, 109–128, Bloomington: Indiana University Press, 2007, 109.

50. Horn, David G., *The Criminal Body: Lombroso and the Anatomy of Deviance,* New York: Routledge, 2003, 80–81.

51. Lombroso and Ferrero, *Criminal Woman,* 143.

52. Ibid., 121–122.

53. Ibid., 123.

54. Ibid., 131–132.
55. Horn, "This Norm Is Not One," 117–118.
56. Tarnovskaia [Tarnowsky], *Étude anthropométrique sur les prostituées et les voleuses*, 97.
57. For an interesting discussion of the collection of crime statistics for Russian women, see Frank, Stephen P., "Narratives within Numbers: Women, Crime and Judicial Statistics in Imperial Russia, 1834–1913," *The Russian Review*, vol. 55, no. 4 (October 1996): 541–566.
58. Lombroso and Ferrero, *Criminal Woman,* 160.
59. Ibid., 166.
60. Ibid., 168.
61. Ibid., 188.
62. Ibid., 198.
63. Ibid., 213 and 240.
64. Lombroso, Cesare, *Crime, Its Causes, and Its Remedies,* translated by Henry P. Horton, London: William Heineman, 1911.
65. Pick, *Faces of Degeneration*, 118–120.
66. Mogilner, "The Empire-Born Criminal," 36–37; 43–44.
67. Pick, *Faces of Degeneration*, 120–121.
68. Gibson, Mary, *Born to Crime: Cesare Lombroso and the Origins of Biological Criminology,* Westport: Praeger, 2002, 82–85.
69. Tarnovskaia, P.N. [Tarnowsky, Pauline], "Criminalité de la femme," in *Congrès international d'athropologie criminelle, Compte-rendu des travaux de la quatrième session tenue à Genève du 24 au 29 août 1896*, Geneva: Georg & Co., 1897, 231–237, https://archive.org/stream/congrsinternat1897cong/congrsinternat-1897cong_djvu.txt.
70. Mazzarello, Paolo, *Il genio e l'alienista. La visita di Lombroso a Tolstoj,* Naples: Bibliopolis, 1998; Nicolosi, "Criminality, Deviance, and Anthropological Diversity," 85–86; Sirotkina, *Diagnosing Literary Genius*, 75–79.
71. Tarnovskaia, P.N., *Zhenshchiny-ubiitsy: Antropologicheskoe issledovanie s 163 risunkami i 8 antropometricheskimi tablitsami,* St. Petersburg: Tovarishchestvo khudozhestvennoi pechati, 1902, III.
72. Ibid., VII.
73. Ibid., 73.
74. Ibid., 73–74.
75. Beer, "Blueprints for Change," 28–29.
76. The Russian (98–99) and French (98–99) texts organize these classifications differently. I have given preference to the French translation as I surmise that Tarnovskaia made the organization of classifications clearer in this later text.
77. Meyer, Adolph, "Les Femmes Homicides by Pauline Tarnowsky," *The Journal of Philosophy, Psychology, and Scientific Methods,* vol. 5, no. 20 (September 24, 1908): 556–557.
78. Goring, Charles, "Review: Recent Criminological Works," *Biometrica,* vol. 7, no. 1/2 (July–October 1909): 231–233.

79. Goring, Charles, *The English Convict: A Statistical Study*, London: Darling and Son, Ltd., 1913.

80. MacDonald, Arthur, "Les Femmes Homicides by Pauline Tarnowsky," *Journal of the American Institute of Criminal Law and Criminology*, vol. 1, no. 4 (November 1910): 666–668.

81. MacDonald, Arthur, *Criminology. With an introduction by Dr. Cesare Lombroso,* New York: Funk & Wagnalls, 1893.

82. J.W.G., "Death of Madame Pauline Tarnowsky," *Journal of the American Institute of Criminal Law and Criminology,* vol. 2, no. 2 (July 1911): 270–271.

83. On the issue of the circular (self-confirming) nature found in the literary and medical narratives of degeneration, see White, Frederick H., "The Danger of Decadence and Degeneration," *Russian Literature* (Elsevier Science BV), volume 92 (August 2017): 49–76; White, Frederick H., *Degeneration, Decadence and Disease in the Russian* fin de siècle. *Neurasthenia in the Life and Work of Leonid Andreev*, Manchester: Manchester University Press, 2014.

WORKS CITED

Beer, Daniel. "Blueprints for Change: The Human Sciences and the Coercive Transformation of Deviants in Russia, 1890–1930." *Osiris*, vol. 22, no. 1 (2007): 26–47.

———. "The Medicalization of Religious Deviance in the Russian Orthodox Church (1880–1905)." *Kritika: Explorations in Russian and Eurasian History*, vol. 5, no. 3 (Summer 2004): 451–482.

———. *Renovating Russia: The Human Sciences and the Fate of Liberal Modernity 1880–1930*. Ithaca: Cornell University Press, 2008.

Bernstein, Laurie. *Sonia's Daughters: Prostitutes and Their Regulation in Imperial Russia.* Berkeley: University of California Press, 1995.

Bialkowski, Zygmunt Ronald. "The Transformation of Academic Criminal Jurisprudence into Criminology in Late Imperial Russia," PhD Dissertation, University of California, Berkeley, Fall 2007.

Biografiia.ru: naibolee polnoe sobraniie biografii. http://www.biografija.ru/. Last accessed February 20, 2021.

Bogdanov, Konstantin. *Vrachi, patsienty, chitateli: Patograficheskie teksty russkoi kul'tury XVIII–XIX vekov.* Moscow: O.G.I., 2005.

Corbin, Alain. *Women for Hire. Prostitution and Sexuality in France after 1850.* Translated by Alan Sheridan. Cambridge: Harvard University Press, 1990.

Dril', Dmitrii. *Maloletnye prestupniki. Etiud po voprosu o chelovecheskoi prestupnosti, ee fektorakh, i sredstvakh bor'by s nei*, 2 vols. Moscow: Tip. A. I. Mamontova i Ko., 1884–1888.

———. *Prestupnost' i prestupniki (Ugolovno-psikhologicheskie etiudy)*. St. Petersburg: Izdanie Ia. Kantorovicha, 1895.

Engelstein, Laura. *The Keys to Happiness. Sex and the Search for Modernity in Fin-de-Siècle Russia.* Ithaca, 1992.

"'Étude anthropométrique sur les prostituées et les voleuses.' By Dr Pauline Tarnowsky. Progrés Mèdical 1889." *The Journal of Mental Science*, no. 157, vol. XXXVII (April 1891): 265–268.

Frank, Stephen P. "Narratives within Numbers: Women, Crime and Judicial Statistics in Imperial Russia, 1834–1913," *The Russian Review*, vol. 55, no. 4 (October 1996): 541–566.

Gibson, Mary. *Born to Crime: Cesare Lombroso and the Origins of Biological Criminology.* Westport: Praeger, 2002. 82–85.

Gilman, Sander L. *Difference and Pathology: Stereotypes of Sexuality, Race and Madness.* Ithaca: Cornell University Press, 1985.

Goring, Charles. "Review: Recent Criminological Works." *Biometrica,* vol. 7, no. 1/2 (July–October 1909): 231–233.

———. *The English Convict: A Statistical Study.* London: Darling and Son, Ltd., 1913.

Hatchen, Elizabeth A. "In Service to Science and Society: Scientists and the Public in Late- Nineteenth-Century Russia." *Osiris*, 2nd Series, vol. 17, Science and Civil Society (2002): 171–209.

Horn, David G. *The Criminal Body: Lombroso and the Anatomy of Deviance.* New York: Routledge, 2003.

———. "This Norm Is Not One: Reading the Female Body in Lombroso's Anthropology." In *Deviant Bodies: Critical Perspectives on Difference in Science and Popular Culture,* edited by Jennifer Terry and Jacqueline Urla, 109–128. Bloomington: Indiana University Press, 2007.

Iudin, T. *Ocherki istorii otechestvennoi psikhiatrii.* Moscow: Medgiz, 1951.

J.W.G. "Death of Madame Pauline Tarnowsky." *Journal of the American Institute of Criminal Law and Criminology,* vol. 2, no. 2 (July 1911): 270–271.

Kowalsky, Sharon A. *Deviant Women.* Dekalb: Northern University Press, 2009.

Lindsey, Edward. "The International Congress of Criminal Anthropology: A Review." *Journal of the American Institute of Criminal Law and Criminology*, vol. 1, no. 4 (November 1910): 578–583.

Lombroso, Cesare. *Crime, Its Causes, and Its Remedies.* Translated by Henry P. Horton. London: William Heineman, 1911.

Lombroso, Cesare and Salvatore Ottolenghi. *La donna delinquente e la prostituta.* Torino: Stamperia dell'unione tip. editrice, 1892.

Lombroso, Cesare and Pauline Tarnowsky. "Fotografie di criminali russe." *Archivio di psichiatria, scienze penali ed antropologia criminale*, volume 14 (1893): 273–275.

Lombroso, Cesare and Gulielmo Ferrero. *Criminal Woman, the Prostitute and the Normal Woman.* Translated and introduced by Nicole Hahn Rafter and Mary Gibson. Durham: Duke University Press, 2004.

———. *Zhenshchina prestupnitsa i prostitutka.* Translated and introduced by Dr. G.I. Gordon. Kiev; Kharkov: F.I. Ioganson, 1897.

MacDonald, Arthur. *Criminology. With an Introduction by Dr. Cesare Lombroso.* New York: Funk & Wagnalls, 1893.

———. "Les Femmes Homicides by Pauline Tarnowsky." *Journal of the American Institute of Criminal Law and Criminology*, vol. 1, no. 4 (November 1910): 666–668.

Mailis, N.P. *Osnovy daktiloskopii. Kurs lektsii.* Moscow: RGUP, 2016.

Mazzarello, Paolo. *Il genio e l'alienista. La visita di Lombroso a Tolstoj.* Naples: Bibliopolis, 1998.

Meyer, Adolph. "Les Femmes Homicides by Pauline Tarnowsky." *The Journal of Philosophy, Psychology, and Scientific Methods,* vol. 5, no. 20 (September 24, 1908): 556–57.

Mogilner, Marina. *Homo Imperii: A History of Physical Anthropology in Russia.* Lincoln: University of Nebraska Press, 2013.

———. "The Empire-Born Criminal. Atavism, Survivals, Irrational Instincts, and the Fate of Russian Imperial Modernity." In *Born to be Criminal.* Edited by Nicolosi and Hartmann, 31–62.

Nicolosi, Riccardo and Anne Hartmann, eds. *Born to be Criminal: The Discourse on Criminality and the Practice of Punishment in Late Imperial Russia and Early Soviet Union. Interdisciplinary Approaches.* Bielefeld: Transcript-Verlag, 2017.

Nicolosi, Riccardo. "Criminality, Deviance, and Anthropological Diversity: Narratives of Inborn Criminality and Atavism in Late Imperial Russia (1880–1900)." In *Born to be Criminal.* Edited by Nicolosi and Hartmann, 85–116.

Pick, Daniel. *Faces of Degeneration: A European Disorder, c. 1848–c. 1918.* Cambridge: Cambridge University Press, 1989.

Rafter, Nicole, ed. *The Origins of Criminology: A Reader.* New York: Routledge, 2009.

Sirotkina, Irina. *Diagnosing Literary Genius. A Cultural History of Psychiatry in Russia, 1880–1930.* Baltimore: The Johns Hopkins University Press, 2002.

Tarnovskaia, P.N. "Antropometricheskie issledovaniia prostitutok, vorovok i zdorovykh krest'ianok-polevykh rabotnits (zasedanie 21 noiabria 1887 g.)." In *Protokoly zasedanii obshchestva psikhiatrov v S.-Peterburge za 1887 god.* St. Petersburg, 1888.

———. [Tarnowsky, Pauline]. "Criminalité de la femme." In *Congrès international d'athropologie criminelle, Compte-rendu des travaux de la quatrième session tenue à Genève du 24 au 29 août 1896.* Geneva: Georg & Co., 1897: 231–237.

———. [Tarnowsky, Pauline]. *Étude anthropométrique sur les prostituées et les voleuses*. Paris: Progrés Mèdical, 1889.

———. "Fisionomie di prostitute russe." *Archivio di psichiatria, scienze penali ed antropologia criminale*, volume 14 (1893): 141–142.

———. [Tarnowsky, Pauline]. *Les femmes homicides.* Paris: F. Alcan, 1908.

———. *Novye raboty po kriminal'noi antropologii. Doklad i sektsii Russkogo Obshchestva okhranenia narodnogo zdravia, 27 dekabria 1891.* St. Petersburg: Tipografiia doma prezreniia maloletnikh bednykh, 1892.

———. "Sur les organes des sens chez les femmes criminelles." In *Actes du troisième congrès international d'anthropologie criminelle tenu a Bruxellesen aout 1892.* Brussels: F. Hayez, 1893: 224–233.

———. *Vorovki (antropologicheskoe issledovanie).* St. Petersburg: Tipografiia doma prezreniia maloletnikh bednykh, 1891.

———. *Zhenshchiny-ubiitsy: Antropologicheskoe issledovanie s 163 risunkami i 8 antropometricheskimi tablitsami.* St. Petersburg: Tovarishchestvo khudozhestvennoi pechati, 1902.

White, Frederick H. "The Danger of Decadence and Degeneration." *Russian Literature* (Elsevier Science BV), volume 92 (August 2017): 49–76.

———. *Degeneration, Decadence and Disease in the Russian* fin de siècle. *Neurasthenia in the Life and Work of Leonid Andreev.* Manchester: Manchester University Press, 2014.

Wolfgang, Marvin E. "Pioneers in Criminology: Cesare Lombroso (1835–1909)." *The Journal of Criminal Law, Criminology, and Police Science,* vol. 52, no. 4 (November–December 1961): 361–391.

Chapter Six

Narrative Medicine in Chekhov and Bulgakov

Melissa L. Miller

In recent years the field of narrative medicine has received particular attention for its call to train physicians to treat their patients as human beings with complex individual stories, as opposed to a strict focus on the discrete symptoms of disease.[1] In doing this, narrative medicine aims not only to validate the experience of the patient, but also to encourage creativity and self-reflection in the physician. Medical schools at leading institutions such as The University of North Carolina at Chapel Hill and New York University, among many others, have introduced courses in narrative medicine into their curricula, while Columbia University, under the leadership of the pioneer in this emerging field, Dr. Rita Charon, has developed a master's program devoted to narrative medicine. These programs feature a multidisciplinary approach that combines the expertise of both clinician and non-clinician faculty, as well as writers and other creative artists, to help train future health professionals to hone their narrative skills in order to deliver personalized and equitable care to their future patients.

But, as I will discuss in this chapter, these ideas are not new or particular to the West, despite the fact that often only Western points of view are discussed in American letters. Though the interdisciplinary field of narrative medicine has its origins in the Anglo-American academic tradition,[2] its core principles have been profoundly shaping the careers and creative output of Russian physician-writers since the nineteenth century. Perhaps the most prominent figure in this category is Anton Chekhov (1860–1904), who both practiced as a physician and was one of Russia's most successful authors and playwrights. While training in the medical faculty at Moscow State University in the early 1880s, he began to write humorous short stories to support himself and his family. Upon graduation, Chekhov practiced medicine formally, first working during the summer as a doctor at a hospital in the provincial town of Voskresensk, and later, at his own practice in Moscow. Though writing soon took precedence—his creative work was what made his reputation and secured his family's long-term comfort—Chekhov never officially turned his back on medicine, continuing to treat both relatives and friends and to provide medical assistance to the communities in which he lived. Regarding the synergetic relationship between literature and medicine, Chekhov brooked no hesitation, as he had been aware of connections between the medical and artistic realms since his university days. While studying under professor G.A. Zakharin (1829–1897), whom Chekhov placed "on a level in medicine with Tolstoy in literature,"[3] the young author learned that no two medical cases, even when the root cause is the very same disease, are ever exactly alike. This scientific approach formed the basis of Chekhov's writing method, for, as leading scholar V. B. Kataev remarks, "individualizing each separate event became one of his basic artistic principles."[4] Chekhov himself, near the end of his life, in the only autobiography he would ever write, declared, "I have no doubt that lectures in the medical sciences had a serious influence on my literary work; they significantly expanded the sphere of my observations, and they enriched me with knowledge, the true value of which for me as a writer can only be understood by one who is themselves a doctor."[5] The most famous example of a Chekhov tale which braids these two themes together is also one of his most autobiographical works, 1889's "A Boring Story." Through the story's hero, a professor of medicine who struggles to come to grips with his own terminal illness, Chekhov demonstrates that true education, both medical and beyond, is imparted not through charts and clinical dissections, but instead lies in the ability to connect with the suffering of a fellow human being, a lesson that the dying physician ironically learns too late. The story has garnered praise both from contemporary physicians, who credit it with possessing "remarkable insight into the psychological problems of academic medicine,"[6] as well as from scholars, such as Donald Rayfield, who rates the form and structure of this "remarkably modern" yet "lyric" tale as "the most satisfying of Chekhov's works."[7]

Beyond the realm of fiction, Chekhov realized in the early 1890s that medical school faculties should include more than the traditional scientific training in subjects such as biology, anatomy, and physiology. Rather, they should also hire literature specialists that could push students to hone their empathetic skills by reading and analyzing fiction. As Cathy Popkin notes, both creative prose and medicine are linked in "their shared concern with access to the pain of others."[8] In this connection, Chekhov proposed himself as the very professor that Moscow University's Medical School needed, a medically informed practitioner of the creative word who could teach his students to harness the power of narrative to facilitate their own future patients' healing. In a letter to his former classmate and prominent neuropathologist G. I. Rossolimo (1860–1928), whose help he sought in securing a faculty position, Chekhov described his teaching methodology in the following way: "If I were a teacher, I would try to draw my audience as deeply as possible into the area of subjective feeling of patients, for I think it would prove really useful to the students."[9] Chekhov also added that he would teach his lectures "as though he were sitting in the examined patient's skin."[10] Undoubtedly, Chekhov's proposal was informed on some level by the fact that he himself had a terminal illness, tuberculosis, and so he had some sense of the value that empathetic doctors could provide to their patients in determining the best course of treatment. Moreover, Chekhov directly acknowledged that one's own personal illness could be a boon to the attending physician, for, as he further confided to Rossolimo, "I, for example, suffer from intestinal catarrh and I understand perfectly what a patient experiences, what kinds of tortures he endures in his soul, and that is something that is rarely clear to a doctor."[11]

Chekhov, however, proved to be too far ahead of his time, institutionally speaking, for Moscow University turned down his request. In response, Chekhov devoted himself to writing an impressive range of stories which fulfilled on the page what Moscow University's medical faculty had denied him in the auditorium. Contemporary scholars and health professionals alike now credit Chekhov's pedagogical approach with having been truly prescient, for it preempted interdisciplinary fields that became popular in the twentieth century, such as the medical humanities and psychosomatic medicine.[12] As literary critic Carl Fisher observes, Chekhov's doctor-written narratives "now seem like standard medical humanities curriculum: representations of doctors and patients, health and illness, aging, death and grieving, and topics related to bodily integrity, psychological wellness, ethics, morality, class, gender, and access issues."[13] Indeed, physician and professor in the Department of Family and Preventative Medicine at UC-San Diego Lawrence Schneiderman made Chekhov's stories a cornerstone of his course on literature and medicine, for "nowhere else in the medical curriculum did [students] confront and discuss the wide array of human concerns raised by Chekhov (and [their] patients)—the deep and painful thoughts and feelings aroused by illness and death, the capriciousness of fate, the unexpected dignity in suffering, the power of simple acts of kindness, and the haunting desires and ambitions we discover in ourselves, sometimes at the worst of times."[14]

As these testimonials suggest, Chekhov's readers have a head-start in integrating their diagnostic and empathetic practices into a cohesive whole. For the remainder of this chapter, I will focus on the work of one of his most famous readers, Mikhail Bulgakov (1891–1940), who, as another physician-cum-author-cum-playwright in the Russian tradition, developed Chekhov's legacy of narrative medicine in his creative prose. In order to demonstrate how Bulgakov's work anticipates both the pleasures, as well as some of the growing pains, that characterize the modern medical humanities, I will draw upon theoretical support from canonical texts on narrative medicine in English. In addition to establishing a relationship between Western medical humanism and Russian literature, which has heretofore been understudied and underrecognized, this approach will also yield new insights into Bulgakov's texts themselves.

Bulgakov was born in 1891 in Kiev, then a part of the Russian Empire. Like Chekhov, Bulgakov grew up in a large, observant Orthodox family. Unlike Chekhov, however, whose father was a merchant and whose grandfather had been a serf, Bulgakov was raised in a decidedly intellectual atmosphere, as his mother was a teacher and his father a professor at the Kiev Theological Academy. While Bulgakov himself, somewhat flippantly, claimed that he became a doctor because he was fascinated by microscopes,[15] it is much more likely that the young man initially chose medicine because several family members were also physicians. Indeed, this kinship influence was strong, for one of Bulgakov's brothers, Nikolai, later became an internationally renowned bacteriologist. Bulgakov studied medicine at Kiev University, and after graduating in 1916, the course of his medical career was charted by the compass of war. Upon graduation, Bulgakov worked for the summer as a Red Cross doctor in Western Ukraine, as part of the tsarist army's effort in World War I. In September of that year, he was posted to a rural hospital in the Smolensk province of Russia, about 250 miles southwest of Moscow, to replace doctors there who had been sent to the front. He remained in the region until February 1918, when he was honorably discharged. He then moved back to Kiev, where he opened a private practice. However, if Bulgakov thought he was returning to a tranquil home life, he was sorely mistaken, for the impending Bolshevik Revolution was to inflict severe consequences on both him and his family. Many of his closest relatives would emigrate to Europe during this time, while Bulgakov himself, as a qualified and experienced physician, was in high demand as each successive government battled for control of the Ukrainian capital during the ensuing Civil War between the Bolshevik Reds and the Tsarist Whites. As a result, Bulgakov was mobilized several times to serve as an army doctor. These experiences provided fertile material for his belletristic works, and after a serious bout with typhus in 1919, Bulgakov formally left his medical practice to become a full-time writer.

When Bulgakov began to publish his first stories, journal editors were struck by how similar his writing style was to Chekhov's. According to Bulgakov's American biographer Ellendea Proffer, editors noted "Bulgakov's speed and seeming ease of composition, comparing it to the young Chekhov's ability to write about whatever his eye chanced to fall upon."[16] The converse was also true, with early Soviet critics faulting Bulgakov for evincing the same perceived lack of a social agenda that they considered to mar Chekhov's work.[17] In addition to referencing Chekhov's stories in his own writing,[18] we know from Bulgakov's personal correspondence that he organized literary evenings featuring Chekhov in his youth, and that he responded particularly strongly to the senior author's stories which explore the aesthetic impact of disease, such as the 1894 story "The Black Monk," which features a prominent scientist who succumbs to mental illness, hallucinating that the titular Black Monk is pursuing him.[19] Many of Bulgakov's most well-known works also feature semi-autobiographical doctors and characters who have the power to heal, such as his novella *Heart of a Dog* (1925) and his full-length novels *White Guard* (1925) and *The Master and Margarita* (1940), among others. In this chapter I will pay particular attention to a collection of Bulgakov's early short stories, titled *A Country Doctor's Notebook* (1925–1927), precisely because it centers on the symbiotic relationship between medicine and writing. As the title implies, this collection follows the intensely personal experiences of a physician who struggles to provide care to an ailing countryside. Similar to Chekhov's works, these tales, too, have been embraced by Western programs in the medical humanities. For example, Lilian Furst, who was Professor Emerita at UNC-Chapel Hill, shared that both her undergraduate students who were headed to medical school, as well as her reading group of health professionals, read and discussed Bulgakov's stories with "ardent enthusiasm."[20]

While on the whole this collection has received less scholarly attention than Bulgakov's more famous novels and plays, it deserves further examination. Ellendea Proffer downplays the significance of the collection, labeling the stories "strikingly un-Bulgakovian in character" and "executed in a style which avoids anything but the most ordinary imagery."[21] Another reason often put forth for the relative neglect of *A Country Doctor's Notebook* is that critics have prized the carnivalesque and supernatural in his later works at the expense of earlier stories, which are supposedly more realistic.[22] However, as modern investigations in narrative medicine elucidate, the process of becoming a qualified and competent doctor is *itself* full of the macabre, the ridiculous, and even the surreal, or to borrow physician-scholar Terrence Holt's term, "the medical sublime."[23] Rita Charon eloquently describes the rupture with everyday reality that the physician-in-training must first undergo and then somehow manage to reconcile themselves to afterward:

> When becoming physicians, young medical students undergo dramatic personal transformations, often in a relatively short time, that render themselves unrecognizable to themselves. To become a person who can dissect a cadaver or peer inside a living human body or inflict pain on another person requires one to turn

> from one's past, during which one did not perform these acts. This inserts an obligatory discontinuity into any medical autobiography.[24]

Relatedly, Holt describes this break in mythopoetic terms, as "an initiation that provides a key by which the initiate learns to understand a new relation to the world. Between the human being who feels a proper loathing and horror of the corpse and all it means and the doctor who will . . . deliberately rebreak a screaming child's arm so that it will heal straight, there must be some division, some lasting estrangement, or else the work will not get done."[25] Bulgakov himself was very much aware of the decidedly *ab*normal nature inherent in real-life medical training, and it is his exploration of precisely how a rational person adapts to these fresh absurdities—the ludicrous pumping of the stomach of a Russian peasant who took ten doses of malaria treatment at once in the interest of modern convenience, the otherworldly yet comical delivery of a newborn on the side of the road by the doctor with his morning shaving cream still covering half his face—that propels the narrative of *A Country Doctor's Notebook* forward. In this way, the medical humanities are able to reveal connections between Bulgakov's earlier and later works that have gone unnoticed.

But first, a note on the text itself. Because these tales were originally released individually in journals from 1925 through 1927, and only later gathered together for publication as a whole, there is some disagreement over whether the collection is a true cycle, especially since there are inconsistencies regarding the unities of time and place. Correspondence with his mother, as well as footnotes to the texts as they were originally published, indicate that Bulgakov had intended to correct these discrepancies and polish the stories into a cohesive work, though he did not get the chance to do so, due to political upheavals and his own premature death.[26] For the purposes of this article, I consider the nine stories that Michael Glenny includes in his translation into English of *A Country Doctor's Notebook* as sufficiently interconnected to merit joint discussion, as they are all based on Bulgakov's background working as a young physician during the Revolution and Civil War in Russia, and feature as their principal subject a newly certified and very insecure medic who only, and even begrudgingly, becomes a capable and effective physician by connecting with his patients and narrating their experiences of illness. As scholar Barbara Henry demonstrates in her discussion of one of the later stories in the collection, as the young doctor matures, "storytelling—as constitutive narrative force and unifying thematic thread in the young doctor stories—saves lives."[27]

This collection is also notable for the fact that all of the stories but one were originally printed in a medical journal titled *The Medical Worker*, which was intended for the continuing education of health professionals, and not in literary magazines for more general readers. In keeping with such a journal's pedagogical mission, *A Country Doctor's Notebook* familiarizes readers with the kinds of highly varied and variable medical emergencies a new doctor would be forced to contend with in the countryside, such as farming and carriage accidents, croup and other illnesses of childhood, syphilis, labor and delivery, as well as all manner of unknown infections. It is telling that the literary device which binds together all the stories of *A Country Doctor's Notebook* as a whole is the metaphor of pitch-black darkness as ignorance, which stands in contrast to the warm light of understanding. Bulgakov's young hero is forced, for example, to undertake delicate medical operations in dark rooms, fields, and embankments during blizzards and gales, during which only the faint light offered by a kerosene lamp or a lone light bulb points the way toward healing knowledge. One of the stories is even titled "Black as Egypt's Night," which in Russian is a folk expression, deriving from Exodus 10:21–23, meaning "pitch-black darkness." This obscurity stands in sharp contrast to the doctor's memories of his medical school days in Moscow, during which the brightly burning electric light imbues every surface—from the "shiny tiled floor" to the "sparkling taps and apparatus everywhere"[28]—with the promise of modern, restorative efficiency. According to Glenny, the ignorance in the collection is that of the uneducated and illiterate Russian peasant, against which Bulgakov's young alter ego must marshal his wits in order to heal the countryside.[29] And indeed, the doctor does have to contend with superstitious mothers and would-be Baba Yagas who would welcome an exorcism with open arms, but who will not allow their babies or grandbabies to receive a life-saving surgical operation; for example, in the story "The Steel Throat," the doctor must perform an emergency tracheotomy so that a young girl will not suffocate to death of diphtheritic croup, in spite of the emphatic protests of her mother and grandmother.

However, at least just as important to the creative struggle and ultimate triumph of the collection as a whole is the ignorance of the young doctor himself. A far greater barrier to healing than any pagan belief the doctor must reason, logic, and even hoodwink away is his own crippling self-doubt and lack of proficiency when it comes to interfacing between his patients' experiences of illness and his knowledge of medicine. The modern medical humanities counts as one of its three main goals the ability to bridge the gulf between science and human experience, and it is precisely this competency that the doctor lacks at the beginning of the collection.[30] As Kalpana Sahni notes, "the constant reference to the doctor's inexperience acts simultaneously as an indirect indictment of the medical institutes which overlooked the practical side of medicine in their courses of study."[31] Over the course of the collection, Bulgakov's doctor beats back the darkness within himself by developing knowledge of his own talents, weaknesses, and techniques, a knowledge he comes to only by transmitting and reflecting on his patients' tales of illness, crisis, and recovery to his readers.

Throughout the collection, Bulgakov's hero addresses his readers directly, in order to relate, and thus to make sense of, that which puzzles and frightens him. In this way, he is constantly, albeit often sarcastically and even reluctantly, reflecting on himself and his practice, which is another one of the chief goals of the medical humanities.[32] Here Bulgakov's narrator is in line with the preeminent physician-scholar working in narrative medicine today, College of Physicians and Surgeons of Columbia University Professor Rita Charon, who writes stories "about patients who trouble or baffle [her]" in order to grow in confidence as a physician and to gain "access to knowledge—about the patient and about [herself]—that would otherwise have remained out of reach."[33] As we will see, Bulgakov ultimately shows the benefits provided by narrative medicine, for we see his young doctor making progress using these very techniques. One medical event that Bulgakov's narrator fears the most, for he reiterates his horror multiple times in several stories across the collection, is having to deliver a baby during a difficult birth. This area is perhaps the darkest region of his ignorance, for he has never attended at a birth himself and has only watched two labor and deliveries, both of which were perfectly normal and complication-free. As a male physician, he also, quite naturally, cannot extrapolate the events and sensations of childbirth from any interior personal experience of his own. It is also worth noting that this was an area of medicine that in general was a point of deep ignorance in the late nineteenth and twentieth centuries, for both men and women have been reluctant to write about childbirth in all of its challenging and visceral detail.[34] In a metafictional way, then, Bulgakov's story also shines a light on this larger information gap, as well.

Bulgakov was an attentive and perceptive reader of his predecessor Chekhov, who famously was fond of saying that a writer who puts a gun into the first act of his play must have it go off by the end.[35] Bulgakov, too, knows that, after so many mentions of childbirth and the dread it induces in his hero, the baby must also, so to speak, fire by the end of the action. Therefore, in a story in the middle of the collection, called "Baptism by Rotation," the physician is forced to attend a young peasant woman who is experiencing a difficult birth. On the surface, this title refers straightforwardly to the fetus, for he is in a position called transverse lie, which Bulgakov has his hero explain in a technical yet approachable way. This position makes vaginal birth impossible, because the baby is lying sideways in the mother's womb. At this time and in this place, performing a Caesarean section would have been unworkable, due to lack of proper training, equipment, and supplies. In this context, in order to correct the position and allow the birth to proceed, the medical professional must manually turn the fetus around by the foot while it is still in the uterus of the mother. Therefore, a rotation is required in order to bring the child into the world.

But this birth story in the young doctor's telling becomes much more than just the clinical diagnosis of the situation given above. Without realizing it himself, the doctor nonetheless shares the details of the labor and delivery with us in a manner that relates his patient's humanity, emphasizing the woman's sympathy-inducing groans and strands of hair that frame her face. He even gives his readers an indication of how severe his patient's pain is—a pain he himself, after all, is unable to comprehend fully and personally—by describing instead her precise physical movements, which consist of her "moaning, stretching herself out, digging her fingers into the bedding and crumpling it up."[36] Finally, once the baby is delivered, the relieved doctor underscores that both the mother and child are alive, healthy, and transported together to the recovery room.

However, in telling his patient's story, the neophyte physician is also confronting his own. Both of these narrative lines merge into each other while he is staring into his patient's anguished face, trying to determine how to proceed in order to deliver her child safely. In this moment, passages from his medical textbooks come flooding back to him, including one in particular where it is written that "a transverse lie is an absolutely inauspicious position."[37] Reflecting on both his medical education and the complicated birth at hand, the doctor realizes that the situation is "absolutely inauspicious" for both him *and* his patients. Thus, the story of delivering his patient's baby, of one body becoming two, becomes the story of his own transformation as well. As the baby struggles to be born, so too do we see Bulgakov's hero struggle to become the kind of physician who is capable of dealing with complex situations. In the beginning of the birth, he is also "stuck," so to speak, without a path forward. In his panic, he flees the operating room for his own, where he becomes engrossed in his textbooks on obstetrics. However, instead of these passages aiding him, they block his progress, because they force him to focus too acutely on discrete, specific symptoms and minute classifications and less on the overall picture. In his own words, his head is in a complete muddle.[38] It is only when he forces himself to stop fixating on technical terms such as "combined version," "bi-polar version," and "external or internal version" that he is able to perform the procedure necessary to turn the fetus and deliver the child.[39] In other words, it is only when he heeds the call of narrative medicine, to focus more on the whole person before him and less on a cluster of symptoms, that he can successfully bring new life into the world. The visceral process of the birth itself solidifies the connection between the newborn and the newly qualified doctor, for the latter makes it a point to tell us readers that they are both covered in pools of the same scarlet blood. By sharing the details of his patient's unique birth story, as well as by reflecting on his own thought process, he shows that Bulgakov's title "Baptism by Rotation" applies to himself too. When he rotates the fetus's foot and pulls him through the mother's birth canal, he also brings *himself* into the world as a more competent physician.

The final image of the story demonstrates the power of focusing on a broader narrative instead of getting caught up in swirls of symptoms, in terms of the kind of deep learning that the theory of narrative medicine tells us leads to better patient care and outcomes. After the birth, the doctor is back in his room, about to go to bed. He notices that his obstetrics textbook is still open, and the very passages that he struggled to comprehend only a few hours earlier are bathed in the glow of his lamp. Only now, after reflecting on his experience of whole childbirth, can he understand perfectly what these texts are trying to communicate, "as though they had been flooded with light."[40] Bulgakov's story left a profound impression on his audience, for, as Milne remarks, "the effectiveness of this device can be demonstrated by the fact that, in Soviet intellectual circles, every parent-to-be knows that a transverse lie is absolutely the worst possible position in which a baby can present itself."[41]

After this incident, the doctor is already a different kind of physician, one who does not need to make excuses to run back to his room to consult his textbooks in order to treat his patients. For example, in the subsequent story "The Starry Rash," Bulgakov begins with the doctor examining a new male patient who is complaining of a sore throat. (Though chaos and confusion bedevil the cycle's timeline, we can suppose with reasonable accuracy that this story takes place after "Baptism by Rotation," for the former takes place in the autumn, while "The Starry Rash" presents the year's first winter snowfall.) This time, the doctor is able not only to recognize the symptoms of syphilis accurately—hoarseness and a white mottled rash that shines forth "like stars in the sky"—but he also has begun to recognize his patients' intrinsic worth as fellow humans, and this realization, in turn, enables him to more effectively prescribe treatment. "A Starry Rash" presents, for the first time in the cycle, the doctor noticing, to his great surprise, "importance and a sense of one's own personal dignity" reflected in his patient's eyes.[42] This revelation, along with his growing ability to empathize with his patients—he bonds with a young female patient by jointly hurling such epithets as "swine" and other abusive names at the "dearest husband" who might have infected her—moves him to fight for those under his care, to obtain scarce equipment and supplies in order to cure them. This growing connection with his patients enables the doctor to save many lives, including those of an entire family, from the ravages of syphilis by the end of the tale. Henry also notes the doctor's increasing self-awareness across the collection as indicative of his personal development, for his "literal capacity for self-reflection" is what separates the mature physician of the later stories from the greenhorn who opened the cycle.[43]

However, *A Country Doctor's Notebook* offers more than the apparently straightforward story of a young physician's development from awkward beginner to confident professional which it might depict on the surface. Perhaps most complex and worthy of further exploration is the collection's second-to-last story, "Morphine," and the ways in which it anticipates some of the modern-day problems associated with narrative medicine. As a discipline, narrative medicine is largely considered to be a positive development, thanks to the fact that it has the potential to forge new paths for wellness, treatment, as well as to deliver higher doctor-patient satisfaction levels and family satisfaction levels.[44] However, some practitioners and scholars, including faculty at the very medical schools that offer degree programs in the medical humanities, have raised certain caveats. As Josephine Ensign, professor of community health at the University of Washington and family nurse practitioner, notes, "current narrative medicine discourse assumes an ideal encounter between an empathetic physician and a cognitively intact, compliant adult patient. What does this mean for providers or for patients who fall outside these parameters?"[45] In other words, can stories from sources that we might be prejudiced against or even consider "damaged" have the power to heal? Do they get listened to or heeded in the same ways that narratives from neurotypical, well-behaved patients do? Is there a way to encourage audiences, in the words of Sayantani DasGupta, physician and faculty member at Columbia's Program in Narrative Medicine, to listen "not only to comfortable stories, or stories of folks who are just like them, but also stories that challenge them, stories that are from the margins, stories that are traditionally silenced"?[46]

Though he was writing a century before Ensign, DasGupta, as well as many others, posed these perceptive questions, Bulgakov, too, considered the potential problems that arise when the narrative is coming from a marginalized source. His autobiographical story "Morphine," based on his own dependence on the drug that, in part, led him to switch his full-time career from medicine to writing, both raises this very problem as well as demonstrates the ultimate merit of such testimony. Reactions to "Morphine" from both Bulgakov's personal acquaintance and critics alike reveal the biases readers have toward storytellers who are broken and undesirable.[47] The topic does not seem to have registered as worthy of literature to Bulgakov's friend

Yury Slezkin, a popular author during the early Soviet period, who dismissed an early draft of the work as being "about some drug addict,"[48] while critic A. Colin Wright disparages the story as "wearisome" and claims that, when it was republished in the literary journal *Russian Thought* many years after Bulgakov's death, a whole page was accidentally left out, but that this omission was not at all noticeable, presumably because the story was too boring to make any impression![49] For her part, Proffer considers the story to end "melodramatically" and as a whole to be "quite badly done."[50] Moreover, in the authoritative study in English of Bulgakov's major works, scholar Lesley Milne devotes a scant half-page to "Morphine," brushing it off as a "somewhat sensational story."[51] However, as I will discuss below, "Morphine" is, both formally and thematically, the most sophisticated piece in the collection, and for this reason it merits further study.

In circumstances that hew uncomfortably close to the modern-day opioid crisis in North America, Bulgakov's tale follows a promising young, yet increasingly mentally unstable, doctor as he succumbs to morphine addiction. This story concerns the young doctor from previous stories, now named Bomgard and posted to a town hospital, and his medical school classmate Dr. Polyakov, who has also been sent to a remote post at a country clinic. But unlike Bomgard, who is able to persevere via a combination of sheer pigheadedness and ironic, self-deprecating humor, Polyakov falls prey to narcosis in his attempts to survive his assignment as an isolated doctor responsible for the health of a rural district's entire population. Critics have often remarked on the fact that, in creating two very similar doctor characters, Bulgakov has essentially fashioned double alter egos for his younger self: the one that is able to survive the turbulent years of internecine strife and would later go on to Moscow to have a career, and the one who was ultimately overwhelmed by the punishing demands placed upon healers in a time of war.[52] We see this dual connection encoded in the names, for together they form an anagram of the author's own surname: Bomgard and Polyakov.[53] Bulgakov is both figures at once, for while he did come through his dangerous rural medical assignments with body and mind more or less intact, Bulgakov the physician ceased to exist, as he quit medicine in favor of writing after he left his final military hospital post for the newly Soviet capital, Moscow.

Written and published last in the cycle, "Morphine" is a frame story told by two distinct yet related narrators, whose five interlocking parts come together to provide a satisfying conclusion to the adventures of the young doctor. Part I is narrated by Bomgard, who, at the beginning of the tale, is able to reflect on the retrospective virtues of his year of trials in the Russian hinterland, now that he is comfortably ensconced in a provincial town, complete with a modern hospital and the luxury of being able to sleep through the night. Part II, however, shows Bomgard feeling a bit guilty that he should be able to enjoy such civilized pleasures, while someone else surely must be taking his place at the backwoods clinic. And indeed, these prophetic thoughts are interrupted by a letter which Bomgard receives from a former classmate, Dr. Polyakov, who now holds his old position. The junior physician begs Bomgard to come at once, for he is gravely ill. Bomgard makes plans to leave, but in Part III, we discover that Bomgard is too late, for Polyakov has already shot himself. His dying body has been brought to Bomgard's gleaming ward, but the surgeons are unable to save him. Before he dies, he gives Bomgard a notebook in which he documented his struggles, so that his friend can "read the story of [his] illness."[54] As will become clear, Polyakov has chosen his recipient specifically because he is gentle and sympathetic, thus demonstrating the power of physician empathy that narrative medicine champions.[55]

Part IV then presents the reader with these notes directly. Spanning a year, the notes chronicle Polyakov's ever more chaotic descent into addiction. While they begin in coherent sentences, there are small signs that the doctor is already troubled, for he speaks of an unidentified wound and displays a clear desire for total emotional isolation. As the entries go on, and the percentages of the injections of his morphine solution tick upward, his grip on reality becomes more and more uncertain. Part V is presented from Bomgard's point of view once again, offering a metaliterary commentary on his motivations for publishing Polyakov's story, which he treats with reverence, noting that it was "given to me as a gift."[56] As a proto-practitioner of narrative medicine, Bomgard preserves and relates Polyakov's diary in full, without any attempts to alter, edit, or streamline his story, despite the fact that the narrative is characterized by derailed trains of thought, hallucinogenic reveries, and strange abbreviations. He does so in accordance with the patient's own wishes, since Polyakov wrote them both to "warn others [to] be careful with white crystals dissolved in twenty-five parts of water" for he "put too much trust in them and they have proved to be [his] downfall," as well as to "warn doctors to be more compassionate towards their patients."[57] While the specifics of the ethical code that health professionals should adhere to when publishing their patients' narratives are still being debated in the contemporary medical community, experts agree that obtaining informed consent from patients and/or their families is paramount.[58] Furthermore, in accordance with Jack Coulehan and Anne Hunsaker Hawkins' observation that patient stories involve more stakeholders than just the author,[59] Bomgard has made sure that releasing the diary will not bring undue pain or embarassment to anyone else, for he has made sure that all other parties described therein are either deceased or now living outside of the Soviet Union, never to return. While Bomgard himself does not presume to know what precise lessons his readers should draw from the diaries of a drug addict, he is confident of the fact that they are, indeed, needed.

In this connection, the framework of narrative medicine can help solve one of the most enduring riddles that "Morphine" poses: since "Morphine" was the very last story in the cycle to be published, why is it the case, as Edythe Haber asks, that "after the author's gradual and painstaking molding of an attractive and admirable persona, he found it so necessary to return to an earlier and sorrier version of self"?[60] In other words, if Bulgakov was able to successfully transition from the Bomgard who survived his medical assignment to an insightful and respected author, why did he feel the need to acquaint readers with his failed alter ego Polyakov? Why dredge up such a painful time in a public forum? Yet, Bulgakov must have had a reason, for his correspondence demonstrates that he faithfully worked and reworked varied drafts of "Morphine" over a period of several years.[61] A possible answer to this conundrum may be found in Holt, who argues that the core purpose of narrative medicine is to "recover a familiarity with, an acceptance of, the essentially fractured nature of our selves and our hearts" so that "we might regain an insight that the empiricist disposition of contemporary medicine, for all its explanatory power, has lost the power to see, to express, or to accept."[62] That is to say, by gathering together these splinters of his former physician's self, by having one incarnation preserve the memory, and thus affirm the intrinsic worth, of a previous incarnation, Bulgakov gives a gift to those who struggle. This portrayal of his own fractured identity shows his readers how, through writing and reading—both, as Holt points out, performative acts[63]—they too can embrace, and even value, their fragmented selves.

NOTES

1. I am grateful to Joe Lenkart and his team at the Summer Research Lab (SRL) at the University of Illinois at Urbana–Champaign for these invaluable references, as well as to SRL for providing the grant funding necessary to pursue this project in Summer 2017. I am also indebted to the National Humanities Center, who provided a generous residency and invaluable research support for this project in Summer 2019.

2. For more on this intellectual tradition see Hilger, Stephanie M., "Introduction: Bridging the Divide Between Literature and Medicine," in *New Directions in Literature and Medicine Studies*, Stephanie M. Hilger, ed., London: Palgrave-Macmillan, 2017, 1–12.

3. Kataev, Vladimir, *If Only We Could Know: An Interpretation of Chekhov*, trans. by Harvey J. Pitcher, Chicago: Ivan R. Dee, 2002, 95.

4. Kataev, *If Only We Could Know*, 95.

5. Quoted from Volume XVI of the Academy Edition of Chekhov's *Complete Works* (*Polnoe sobranie sochinenii v 18 tomakh*, Moscow: Nauka, 1974–1983), 271. The translation is my own.

6. Carter, Richard, MD, "Anton P. Chekhov, MD (1860–1904): Dual Medical and Literary Careers," *The Annals of Thoracic Surgery: The Official Journal of The Society of Thoracic Surgeons and The Southern Thoracic Surgical Association*, 61 (1996): 1557–1563, 1560.

7. Rayfield, Donald, *Understanding Chekhov: A Critical Study of Chekhov's Prose and Drama*, Madison: University of Wisconsin Press, 1999, 70, 68. For more on medical issues in "A Boring Story," see, for example, Flath, Carol, "The Limits to the Flesh: Searching for the Soul in Chekhov's 'A Boring Story,'" *Slavic and East European Journal* 41.2 (1997): 271–286; and Gatrall, Jefferson J.A., "The Paradox of Melancholy Insight: Reading the Medical Subtext in Chekhov's 'A Boring Story,'" *Slavic Review* 62.2 (2003): 258–277.

8. Popkin, Cathy, "'A Talent for Humanity': Teaching Chekhov and the Medical Humanities," in *Approaches to Teaching the Works of Anton Chekhov*, Michael C. Finke and Michael Holquist, eds. New York: The Modern Language Association of America, 2016. 151–162, 151.

9. Rossolimo, G.I., "Vospominaniia o Chekhove," in *A.P. Chekhov v vospominaniiakh sovremennikov*, N.I. Gitovich, ed. Moscow: Khudozhestvennaia literatura, 1986, 428–438, 436.

10. Gitovich, N.I., ed., *Letopis' zhizni i tvorchestva A.P. Chekhova,* Moscow: Khudozhestvennaia literatura, 1955, 587.

11. Rossolimo, "Vospominaniia o Chekhove," 436.

12. See, for example, Carter, "Anton P. Chekhov, MD (1860–1904): Dual Medical and Literary Careers"; Finke, Michael, "Heal Thyself, Hide Thyself: Why Did Chekhov Ignore His TB?," in *Chekhov the Immigrant: Translating a Cultural Icon*, Michael C. Finke and Julie de Sherbinin, eds., Bloomington, Indiana: Slavica, 2007, 285–297; Finke, Michael and Richard Kahn, MD, moderators, "Seminar on Anton Chekhov and the Medical Humanities: A Discussion of Selected Chekhov Stories," in *Chekhov the Immigrant: Translating a Cultural Icon*, Michael C. Finke and Julie de Sherbinin, eds., Bloomington, Indiana: Slavica, 2007, 319–336.

13. Fisher, Carl, "Doctor-Writers: Anton Chekhov's Medical Stories," in *New Directions in Literature and Medicine Studies*, Stephanie M. Hilger, ed. London: Palgrave-Macmillan, 2017, 377–396, 377.

14. Schneiderman, L.J., "The Good Doctor: The Literature and Medicine of Anton Chekhov (And Others)," *Family Medicine* 33.1 (2001): 11–13, 12.

15. Quoted in Lakshin's introduction to Bulgakov, Mikhail, *Izbrannia proza*, Moscow: Khudozhestvennaia literatura, 1966, 5.

16. Proffer, Ellendea, *Mikhail Bulgakov: Life and Work*. Ann Arbor, Michigan: Ardis, 1984, 66.

17. See Sahni, Kalpana, *A Mind in Ferment*, Atlantic Highlands, New Jersey: Humanities Press, 1986, 113.

18. For example, one of the stories in *A Country Doctor's Notebook*, "The Vanishing Eye," is explicitly in dialogue with Chekhov's story "The Surgery." See Henry,

Barbara, "Bulgakov's Young Doctor in the Land of the Dead," *The Russian Review* 77 (July 2018): 411–426, 424.

19. Wright, A. Colin, *Mikhail Bulgakov: Life and Interpretations*, Toronto: University of Toronto Press, 1978, 19; Proffer, *Bulgakov: Life and Work*, 341.

20. Furst, Lilian R., "Recognizing Mikhail Bulgakov's *A Country Doctor's Notebook*," *Symposium* 58 (Fall 2004): 167–177, 168.

21. Proffer, *Bulgakov: Life and Work*, 92.

22. See, for example, Furst, "Recognizing Mikhail Bulgakov's *A Country Doctor's Notebook*," 167.

23. Holt, Terrence E., "Narrative Medicine and Negative Capability," *Literature and Medicine* 23, no. 2 (2004): 318–333, 325.

24. Charon, Rita, "Narrative Medicine: Form, Function, and Ethics," *Annals of Internal Medicine* 134 (2001): 83–87, 84.

25. Holt, "Narrative Medicine and Negative Capability," 328.

26. See Bulgakov's letter to his mother of November 17, 1921, in Curtis, J. A. E., *Manuscripts Don't Burn: Mikhail Bulgakov: A Life in Letters and Diaries*, Woodstock, New York: The Overlook Press, 1992, 38; and Milne, Lesley, *Mikhail Bulgakov: A Critical Biography*, New York: Cambridge UP, 1990, 125–126.

27. Henry, "Bulgakov's Young Doctor in the Land of the Dead," 423.

28. All quotations from the stories in *A Country Doctor's Notebook* come from Volume 3 of Bulgakov's definitive *Collected Works*, titled *Sobranie sochinenii v desiati tomakh,* Moscow: Golos, 1995. Citations from this work will be given as *Sobranie sochinenii* plus the appropriate page numbers. All translations from the Russian are my own unless otherwise indicated. *Sobranie sochinenii*, 313.

29. See Glenny's Introduction to Bulgakov, Mikhail, *A Country Doctor's Notebook*, translated by Michael Glenny, New York: Vintage, 2010, 8–9.

30. Cole, Thomas R., Nathan S. Carlin, and Ronald A. Carson, *Medical Humanities: An Introduction,* New York: Cambridge University Press, 2015, 9.

31. Sahni, *A Mind in Ferment*, 33.

32. For more on these goals, see pages 1–18 of Cole, Carlin, and Carson, *Medical Humanities: An Introduction*.

33. Charon, "Narrative Medicine: Form, Function, and Ethics," 84.

34. For more on childbirth in Russian literature, see Maguire, Muireann, "Dostoevsky and the Politics of Parturition: Childbirth as Political Motif in *Demons,*" *Modern Languages Open* [Online], 0.1 (2014): n. pag., Web January 12, 2017; and Miller, Melissa, "'The Name-Day Party': Reconceiving Childbirth in Chekhov and Tolstoy," *The Slavic and East European Journal* 61.4 (2017): 737–754.

35. Reported in Gurliand, I. Ia., "Vospominaniia ob A.P. Chekhove," *Teatr i iskusstvo*, no. 28, July 11, 1904, p. 521.

36. *Sobranie sochinenii,* 312.

37. *Sobranie sochinenii,* 314.

38. *Sobranie sochinenii,* 316.

39. *Sobranie sochinenii,* 316–317.

40. *Sobranie sochinenii,* 319.

41. Milne, *Mikhail Bulgakov: A Critical Biography*, 132.

42. *Sobranie sochinenii,* 343.
43. Henry, "Bulgakov's Young Doctor in the Land of the Dead," 417.
44. See, for example, Charon, Rita, "Literature and Medicine: Origins and Destinies," *Academic Medicine* 75 (2000): 23–27; Charon, "Narrative Medicine: Form, Function, and Ethics"; and Perry, Mark, Nicola Maffulli, Suzy Willson, and Dylan Morrissey, "The Effectiveness of Arts-based Interventions in Medical Education: A Literature Review," *Medical Education* 45 (2011): 141–148.
45. Ensign, Josephine, "The Problem(s) With Narrative Medicine," *Medical Margins: Josephine Ensign on Health Humanities, Policy, Nursing*, Blog post from July 16, 2014, https://josephineensign.com/2014/07/16/the-problems-with-narrative-medicine/. Last accessed August 2, 2019.
46. DasGupta, Sayantani, "Narrative Medicine, Narrative Humility: Listening to the Streams of Stories," *Creative Nonfiction* 52 (Summer 2014), Online journal, no pagination, https://www.creativenonfiction.org/online-reading/narrative-medicine-narrative-humility. Last accessed August 2, 2019.
47. Sympathetic representation of those dependent on drugs is still officially taboo in Russia. For example, on August 19, 2019, the online media outlet *Meduza* reported that Roskomnadzor, Russia's media regulation and censorship agency, demanded that *Meduza* redact an article on drug use because it containted information "intended to cause the target audience to form a positive impression of individuals who produce, process, and use narcotic substances." https://meduza.io/en/news/2019/08/19/russian-censors-tell-meduza-to-redact-article-on-drug-use?fbclid=IwAR17FTy-tedP4671L59eqs35YHyeCEXhVgqbjXD_adHN7ZRz64DrirhZAgI. Last accessed February 20, 2021.
48. Quoted in Haber, Edythe C., *Mikhail Bulgakov: The Early Years*, Cambridge: Harvard UP, 1998, 34.
49. Wright, *Mikhail Bulgakov: Life and Interpretations*, 14.
50. Proffer, *Bulgakov: Life and Work*, 95.
51. Milne, *Mikhail Bulgakov: A Critical Biography,* 137.
52. See, for example, Haber, *Mikhail Bulgakov: The Early Years,* 130. For a fascinating interpretation of Bulgakov's hero(es) as undergoing a katabatic journey to the underworld, see Henry, "Bulgakov's Young Doctor in the Land of the Dead."
53. This quote is reported by Gourg in Milne, Lesley, *Bulgakov: The Novelist-Playwright*, New York: Routledge, 1996, 108.
54. *Sobranie sochinenii,* 427.
55. For more on how physician empathy can encourage patients to share their stories, see Cole, Carlin, and Carson, *Medical Humanities: An Introduction,* 221–224.
56. *Sobranie sochinenii,* 448.
57. *Sobranie sochinenii,* 427; 437.
58. See, for example, Charon, "Narrative Medicine: Form, Function, and Ethics," and Coulehan, Jack and Anne Hunsaker Hawkins, "Keeping Faith: Ethics and the Physician-Writer," *Annals of Internal Medicine* 139 (2003): 307–311.
59. Coulehan and Hawkins, "Keeping Faith: Ethics and the Physician-Writer," 307.
60. Haber, *Mikhail Bulgakov: The Early Years*, 132.

61. Bulgakov began what would eventually become "Morphine," a draft of a novel then called *The Ailment* (*Nedug*), while he was living in Kiev during the period of 1919–1921. For an account of the history of the creation of "Morphine," see Yanovskaya, L., *Tvorcheskiy put' Mikhaila Bulgakova*, Moscow: Sovetskiy pisatel', 1983, 83–88.

62. Holt, "Narrative Medicine and Negative Capability," 330.

63. Holt, "Narrative Medicine and Negative Capability," 330.

WORKS CITED

Bulgakov, Mikhail. *A Country Doctor's Notebook*. Translated by Michael Glenny. New York: Vintage, 2010.

Bulgakov, Mikhail. *Izbrannia proza*. Moscow: Khudozhestvennaia literatura, 1966.

Bulgakov, Mikhail. *Sobranie sochinenii v desiati tomakh*. Moscow: Golos, 1995.

Carter, Richard, MD. "Anton P. Chekhov, MD (1860–1904): Dual Medical and Literary Careers." *The Annals of Thoracic Surgery: The Official Journal of The Society of Thoracic Surgeons and The Southern Thoracic Surgical Association*, 61 (1996): 1557–1563.

Charon, Rita. "Literature and Medicine: Origins and Destinies." *Academic Medicine* 75 (2000): 23–27.

Charon, Rita. "Narrative Medicine: Form, Function, and Ethics." *Annals of Internal Medicine* 134 (2001): 83–87.

Chekhov, Anton. *Polnoe sobranie sochinenii v 18 tomakh*. Moscow: Nauka, 1974–83.

Cole, Thomas R., Nathan S. Carlin, and Ronald A. Carson. *Medical Humanities: An Introduction.* New York: Cambridge University Press, 2015.

Coulehan, Jack and Anne Hunsaker Hawkins. "Keeping Faith: Ethics and the Physician-Writer." *Annals of Internal Medicine* 139 (2003): 307–311.

Curtis, J.A.E. *Manuscripts Don't Burn: Mikhail Bulgakov: A Life in Letters and Diaries*. Woodstock, New York: The Overlook Press, 1992.

DasGupta, Sayantani. "Narrative Medicine, Narrative Humility: Listening to the Streams of Stories." *Creative Nonfiction* 52 (Summer 2014). Online journal, no pagination. https://www.creativenonfiction.org/online-reading/narrative-medicine-narrative-humility. Last accessed August 2, 2019.

Ensign, Josephine. "The Problem(s) With Narrative Medicine." *Medical Margins: Josephine Ensign on Health Humanities, Policy, Nursing*. Blog post from July 16, 2014. https://josephineensign.com/2014/07/16/the-problems-with-narrative-medicine/. Last accessed August 2, 2019.

Finke, Michael. "Heal Thyself, Hide Thyself: Why Did Chekhov Ignore His TB?" In *Chekhov the Immigrant: Translating a Cultural Icon*. Michael C. Finke and Julie de Sherbinin, eds. Bloomington, Indiana: Slavica, 2007. 285–297.

Finke, Michael. *Seeing Chekhov: Life and Art*. Ithaca: Cornell UP, 2005.

Finke, Michael and Richard Kahn, MD, moderators. "Seminar on Anton Chekhov and the Medical Humanities: A Discussion of Selected Chekhov Stories." In *Chek-*

hov the Immigrant: Translating a Cultural Icon. Michael C. Finke and Julie de Sherbinin, eds. Bloomington, Indiana: Slavica, 2007. 319–336.

Fisher, Carl. "Doctor-Writers: Anton Chekhov's Medical Stories." In *New Directions in Literature and Medicine Studies*. Stephanie M. Hilger, ed. London: Palgrave-Macmillan, 2017. 377–396.

Flath, Carol. "The Limits to the Flesh: Searching for the Soul in Chekhov's 'A Boring Story.'" *Slavic and East European Journal* 41.2 (1997): 271–286.

Furst, Lilian R. "Recognizing Mikhail Bulgakov's *A Country Doctor's Notebook*." *Symposium* 58 (Fall 2004): 167–177.

Gatrall, Jefferson J.A. "The Paradox of Melancholy Insight: Reading the Medical Subtext in Chekhov's 'A Boring Story.'" *Slavic Review* 62.2 (2003): 258–277.

Gitovich, N.I., ed. *Letopis' zhizni i tvorchestva A.P. Chekhova*. Moscow: Khudozhestvennaia literatura, 1955.

Gurliand, I. Ia. "Vospominaniia ob A.P. Chekhove." *Teatr i iskusstvo*, no. 28, July 11, 1904, p. 521.

Haber, Edythe C. *Mikhail Bulgakov: The Early Years*. Cambridge: Harvard UP, 1998.

Henry, Barbara. "Bulgakov's Young Doctor in the Land of the Dead." *The Russian Review* 77 (July 2018): 411–426.

Hilger, Stephanie M. "Introduction: Bridging the Divide Between Literature and Medicine." In *New Directions in Literature and Medicine Studies*. Stephanie M. Hilger, ed. London: Palgrave-Macmillan, 2017. 1–12.

Holt, Terrence E. "Narrative Medicine and Negative Capability." *Literature and Medicine* 23, no. 2 (2004): 318–333.

Kataev, Vladimir. *If Only We Could Know: An Interpretation of Chekhov*. Trans. by Harvey J. Pitcher. Chicago: Ivan R. Dee, 2002.

Maguire, Muireann. "Dostoevsky and the Politics of Parturition: Childbirth as Political Motif in *Demons*." *Modern Languages Open* [Online], 0.1 (2014): n. pag., Web January 12, 2017.

Miller, Melissa. "'The Name-Day Party': Reconceiving Childbirth in Chekhov and Tolstoi.'" *Slavic and East European Journal* 61.4 (2017): 714–731.

Milne, Lesley. *Bulgakov: The Novelist-Playwright*. New York: Routledge, 1996.

Milne, Lesley. *Mikhail Bulgakov: A Critical Biography*. New York: Cambridge UP, 1990.

Perry, Mark, Nicola Maffulli, Suzy Willson, and Dylan Morrissey. "The Effectiveness of Arts-based Interventions in Medical Education: A Literature Review." *Medical Education* 45 (2011): 141–148.

Popkin, Cathy. "'A Talent for Humanity': Teaching Chekhov and the Medical Humanities." In *Approaches to Teaching the Works of Anton Chekhov*. Michael C. Finke and Michael Holquist, eds. New York: The Modern Language Association of America, 2016. 151–162.

Proffer, Ellendea. *Mikhail Bulgakov: Life and Work*. Ann Arbor, Michigan: Ardis, 1984.

Rayfield, Donald. *Understanding Chekhov: A Critical Study of Chekhov's Prose and Drama*. Madison: University of Wisconsin Press, 1999.

Rossolimo, G. I. "Vospominaniia o Chekhove." In *A.P. Chekhov v vospominaniiakh sovremennikov*. N. I. Gitovich, ed. Moscow: Khudozhestvennaia literatura, 1986. 428–438.

"Russian Censors Tell 'Meduza' to Redact Article on Drug Use." *Meduza*. https://meduza.io/en/news/2019/08/19/russian-censors-tell-meduza-to-redact-article-on-drug-use?fbclid=IwAR17FTytedP4671L59eqs35YHyeCEXhVgqbjXD_adHN7Z-Rz64DrirhZAgI. Last accessed February 20, 2021.

Sahni, Kalpana. *A Mind in Ferment*. Atlantic Highlands, New Jersey: Humanities Press, 1986.

Schneiderman, L.J. "The Good Doctor: The Literature and Medicine of Anton Chekhov (And Others)." *Family Medicine* 33.1 (2001): 11–13.

Wright, A. Colin. *Mikhail Bulgakov: Life and Interpretations*. Toronto: University of Toronto Press, 1978.

Yanovskaya, L. *Tvorcheskiy put' Mikhaila Bulgakova*. Moscow: Sovetskiy pisatel', 1983.

Chapter Seven

Social Cataclysm through the Doctor's Eyes

Vikentii Veresaev's The Deadlock[1] *as Diagnostic Narrative*

Natalia Vygovskaia

Medicine and literature in the works of Vikentii Veresaev (1867-1945) are intertwined. As Veresaev wrote in his memoirs, he decided to become a doctor because it would help him to become a good writer. Being timid, he hoped to learn more about the intimate side of human nature through the doctor-patient relationship. What he found in common between a doctor and a writer is that both study human bodies and their behavior, the state of being healthy and ill.[2] As the doctor tends to assign each case to a larger group with similar symptoms to diagnose and cure the disease, the writer, from Veresaev's point of view, tells the stories of individuals that illustrate the gravest social problems of his time, looking for solutions to correct them. And hence the mission of the writer: to unveil and vocalize social ills.

Veresaev's fascination with the social aspect of the literary and medical profession can be partly explained by his father, who was also a physician and was engaged in various social activities. In addition to being a general practitioner, his father opened a hospital, organized a sanitary commission, and founded the committee of medics in Tula, a little town over a hundred miles away from Moscow. Additionally, one should keep in mind that after the Emancipation Reform of 1861 the medical profession began to be considered one of the noblest and most socially significant occupations in the Russian Empire. Young people dreaming of changing the world for the better wanted to cure and educate those who previously did not have any access to professional medical assistance.[3] Multiple epidemics of cholera and typhus contributed to the professionalization of the medical field. Physicians collaborated with central and local governments,[4] helping to implement public health policies and educational initiatives in rural areas.[5] Based on material from *Vrach*,[6] the most influential medical journal of the day, doctors may be characterized as the most unified and progressive group of the Russian intelligentsia at that time: as a whole they condemned duels; established a Court of Honor to settle disputes between colleagues; defended the abolition of capital and corporal punishment; raised questions about doctor-patient confidentiality; claimed that healthcare should be a basic human right and that doctors should prioritize their patients' needs over career-driven ambition; deemed sexism unacceptable in medical education; and negotiated the improvement of sanitary conditions for workers, peasants, students, and schoolchildren. Treating all patients regardless of their social status (and free of charge if they could not afford it) was commonly accepted behavior among physicians who dealt on a daily basis with poverty and work-related injuries under the Tsarist regime. In such a context, Veresaev's works exemplify the values and concerns of the medical community.

One may trace the tendency of the educated class to use medical terms for social critique in the Russian first psychological novel *A Hero of Our Time* (1840) by Mikhail Lermontov (1814–1841). In the Foreword the narrator specifies the role of his writing as a diagnostic method to uncover social ills.[7] In the 1850s, the so-called critical realism writers[8] created a genre of physiological sketches, in which they raised their concerns about inequality and the position of the unprivileged class (for example, Dmitrii Grigorovich (1822-1900) and Aleksei Pisemskii (1821-1881)). The language of fiction was conceived as powerful rhetorical artillery, calling for immediate ameliorative action.

This puts Vikentii Veresaev in dialogue with the Russian intelligentsia[9] who would be willing to change the current social order, eventually taking political measures. Marina Mogilner in her thorough study of the nihilistic groups of the late nineteenth and early twentieth centuries calls them "Underground Russia"[10] and argues that writers and poets who belonged to this group saw themselves as mythological heroes, martyrs, and warriors of revolution. Their biographies, saturated with arrests, exile, escape, and struggle, served as role models for young intellectuals. In its extreme form, the urgent need for change resulted in terrorist attacks and the propagation of the ideas of revolution. However, despite his sympathy for socialism, and later Marxism, Veresaev seems to eschew political radicalization. And even when the medical community became politically engaged,[11] Veresaev would not share its revolutionary spirit. On the contrary, his *Notes of a Doctor* (1900) evoked so much criticism[12] in large part because what Veresaev attempted to achieve in problematizing medical ethics was the de-heroization of the medical profession, as well as of the messianic role of doctors who battled against the state for the public good.

In his *Notes*, Veresaev is particularly sensitive to medical malpractice. He scrupulously collects examples of violations of patients' rights, drawing on tiny details. For instance, he points to the poor, who are unable to make decisions regarding the autopsy and burial of their loved ones, because they are patients at a university clinic and their wishes do not count. He also disapproves of experiments on terminally ill patients and reveals the ambiguity of nudity in the examination room. In all facets of the doctor-patient relationship he highlights neglect of the patient's needs, and one may argue that through the same lens he views the reality of the Civil War in his novel *The Deadlock* (1922), in which victims of violence play a critical role in the subsequent suffering of patients. In his *Notes*, Veresaev writes about ethical topics from the perspective of a materialist. For him, human tragedies are caused by randomness and chance. The most illustrative example is a life-threatening disease, striking patients unexpectedly. Rough, enormous, and mighty life[13] does its cruel work, while medicine is still far from understanding its nature. Veresaev talks about the totality of pain that constitutes the essence of human existence. It is unsurprising, therefore, that, in his novel, the writer examined the Civil War as a similar random phenomenon, being able to discern the universality of human suffering caused by social cataclysm, and therefore aspiring to reconcile both sides of the conflict.

Like many of his contemporaries, Veresaev hoped to improve social conditions, and for that reason, he supported the Bolsheviks when the October Revolution broke out. In 1918, Veresaev and his wife left for Koktebel (a town in South-Eastern Crimea) and were planning to stay at their dacha for three months. However, due to the Civil War, their initial three months' stay turned into three years. Veresaev witnessed how the Crimean Peninsula passed through several hands. He was robbed by the Reds (the Bolsheviks) and arrested by the Whites (anti-communist forces). He worked as a physician and accepted eggs and lard as payment for his job. In April of 1919, he was elected the head of the Literature and Arts Department in the Collegium of Public Education in Feodosiya.[14]

The Deadlock is based on Veresaev's everyday experiences. It was an immediate response to the events after the Bolsheviks came to power and presents a written testimony, which was quite different from those penned by his contemporaries. The Civil War is often shown in the literature of that period as the end of civilization, the coming of the time of original creation, the Apocalypse, a mythological battle between the old and the new world, or a heroic epic tale.[15] This imagery does not allow for a dialogue between the two sides of the conflict to take place, because in the imagination of the modernist and the Red writers, the Bolsheviks were purely symbolic. They are not portrayed as human beings. Characters turn into puppets, dolls, icons, and depersonalized disastrous forces, moving to another plane of poetics. Lacking psychological personality traits, they become de-humanized, acquiring instead religious, mythological, folkloric, and/or heroic connotations. *The Deadlock* showcases a distinct response to revolution. Quite uncommonly for the narratives of the 1920s, which scholars identify as modernist novels and autobiography, or early socialist realism writings, Veresaev's text follows the Russian tradition of the psychological novel. It includes traditional characters' biographies, the description of their feelings and thoughts, symbolic seaside landscapes mirroring their mental states, multiple dialogues, and the description of external and internal spaces, where the most violent scenes take place.

The Deadlock is a novel about a doctor's family attempting to survive amid the chaos of the Civil War. The story begins with the Bolsheviks entering Armatluk, a little town near Koktebel. They start the process of the confiscation of houses and valuables from the bourgeoise[16] and the redistribution of the confiscated "wealth," accompanied by arrests and shootings. In addition to the Bolsheviks, there are bands of rebels associated with the Ukrainian anarchist Nestor Makhno harassing neighborhoods. The family patriarch, Doctor Sartanov, is arrested and later pardoned because his nephew works in the Commissariat. His daughter Katia, the main protagonist, gets a job in the public education center and is then arrested but soon released for the same reason. Katia's sister Vera is executed by the White officers, while her mother dies from a stray bullet fired by drunken soldiers. Father and daughter search for a new stability after the October Revolution, which ends in a deadlock because Doctor Sartanov dies of depression, having lost his wife and daughter and traumatized by a mock execution, and Katia (and this is the last line of the novel) disappears "nobody knows where"—a symbolic indication of her disorientation in the new world.[17]

The history of the novel's reception illustrates its distinctiveness. Veresaev had read some excerpts of it to the members of the first Politburo, founded in 1917 to manage the Bolshevik Revolution. As he later wrote in his memoirs, Lev Kamenev (1883–1936), one of its seven members, was against publishing it, but Felix Dzerzhinsky (1877–1926), the Director of the Secret Police, surprisingly defended the novel. However, even final approval to publish the text did not save it from Soviet censorship and publication delays.[18] As William Chamberlin notes in his article about the tragedy of the Russian intelligentsia, Veresaev, whom he had the privilege of knowing personally, mentioned that high-ranking Communist sources promised that the novel would receive great official acclaim if Veresaev "would make Katia become a Communist in the end."[19] Although Katia did accept the Bolshevik regime as a better alternative to Tsarism and the Provisional Government, her experience of the Civil War and war-related violence shatters her beliefs and threatens her identity.

At first glance, one may look at the novel as fictionalized reportage which highlights real-life experiences during the Civil War. However, I would not suggest reading the novel as a journalistic piece, but rather as a diagnostic narrative that enables us to see a more complex formal structure and interpretative potentiality. In the medical humanities, the theory of narratology is mainly used to incorporate narratives about patients into the traditional domain of literature. For example, Thomas Laqueur claimed that such distinct texts as the autopsy, the clinical report, and the realist novel may be unified by so-called *humanitarian* narratives,[20] because all of these pieces contain details about the suffering bodies of others that engender compassion. In such narratives, the detailed description of the body is "the common locus of understanding and sensibility."[21] One may refer to *The Deadlock* as a humanitarian narrative in the sense that the writer intends to evoke an empathetic response from the reader when he describes, for example, acts of physical violence toward the most vulnerable members of the community, such as a priest or a young woman. However, it does not seem sufficient for understanding the author's method. I call this method of narration *diagnostic* not only because of Veresaev's medical education but also because his main protagonist investigates the root of violence in Russian society, employing strategies of doctor-patient communication. When Arthur Kleimann claims in his seminal work that in narrating illness there is always culture that fills the space between "the immediate embodiment of sickness as physiological process and its mediated experience as human phenomenon—for example, as an alienated part of body-self, as a vehicle for transcendence,"[22] I suggest that we could draw another conclusion from the same line of reasoning which is applicable to *The Deadlock*, as well. Literature as a part of culture fills the space between the physiology of violence understood as a contagious disease and its mediated experience as a communication system, in which "the body-self is an organic part of sociocentric world."[23]

The central issue in *The Deadlock* is the normalization of violence. Like a doctor dealing with a yet-undiagnosed disease would examine his patients' symptoms, Veresaev collects these from multiple conversations. Katia and Doctor Sartanov talk to landowners, peasants, workers, soldiers, sailors, and officers of the Cheka. In each conversation, they ask questions and record responses about the nature of class hatred and the new political system. It bears a resemblance to the way Veresaev describes a doctor diagnosing a patient in *Notes*. He asks them lots of questions, and their answers "show the entire life of the sick organism unlike the healthy one."[24] Veresaev's contemporary Dmitrii Merezhkovskii in the 1910 miscellany titled *Sick Russia* also diagnoses state-run violence as a universal condition, but emphasizes its chronic, undetectable nature: "Legalized violence for us is almost impalpable because it is too common . . . this bloodshed is as painless as the blood circulating through one's veins."[25] Unlike Merezhkovskii's fatal diagnosis, Veresaev explores the unknown grounds of the Civil War, hoping to find treatment.[26]

What the dialogues reveal is that the White and the Red sides both view Bolshevism, first of all, as a destructive force. A peasant girl named Uliasha, a supporter of Bolshevism, understands it as "pillaging dachas" because, in her own words, "the gentry does nothing but sunbathe and pick flowers" and their wealth should belong to their servants who do the hard physical work. Dmitrii, Professor Dmitrevskii's son, who joins the White Army, says that the Bolsheviks are cruel and grabby barbarians who destroy civilization. For the aristocracy, the root of the violence is the atheism propagated by the Reds. The priest Zlatoverkhovnikov calls the Bolsheviks wild beasts who are unable to pay respect to the dead, as "they rush to the graves, dig up the bodies and mutilate them."[27] Around the same time, Ivan Bunin in his diary wrote about a similar feeling of outrage that he experienced, when he learned about the Bolsheviks digging trenches near the Kremlin wall to bury dead bodies without last rites or headstones.[28] In her sociological study of Soviet norms and abnormalities in the 1920s and 1930s, Natalia Lebina speaks about the introduction of new norms for funeral services which primitivized long-standing farewell rituals. What priest Zlatoverkhovnikov and Bunin both consider a blasphemy, demonizing the Bolsheviks, was one of the first governmental steps to handle the increased mortality rate and to deprive the Orthodox Church of its spiritual authority. The 1917 decree of the Russian Social Democratic Labor Party required churches to transfer death, birth, and marriage records to local committees. The burning of corpses was part of their anti-religious campaign, and the new political leaders called the crematorium (although the first one was not built until 1927) the "department of godlessness."[29] In this respect, the treatment of the dead becomes a symbolic representation of how the existence of personal memory and selfhood was threatened by bureaucratic institutions. Veresaev's reference to priest Zlatoverkhovnikov indicates the utmost degree of normalization of violence when the official policy enforces the acceleration of collective amnesia and reduces the deceased to a purely material substance.

However, unlike Uliasha, Dmitrii, and the priest, the main protagonist Katia does not see the Bolsheviks as barbarians. For her, the people she talks with are suffering individuals enduring hard times of poverty and uncertainty. Like a doctor trying to find some healthy signs in a sick body which could give hope of a quick recovery, Katia can spot humanizing little details that show the non-violent side of her interlocutors. The high-ranking Cheka officer Voron'ko laughs so sincerely that his eyes fill with tears; sailors and soldiers breaking into houses on confiscation raids suddenly smile back; Uliasha, who approves of the robberies, is described as a pretty girl with blushing cheeks.

One might then wonder whether for Veresaev these conversations have any healing power besides diagnostics. The answer is two-fold. Conversations do function as therapeutic in that they resist the propaganda of extermination when the interlocutors begin to see each other as representatives of one community, as brothers and sisters. For instance, in Katia's conversation with the sailors, Katia's opponent uses the popular propaganda expression "callous hands" (*mozolistye ruki*) trying to prove that having been born to a peasant family, he is more hardworking than she. They end up comparing the number of calluses on their palms, and Katia wins. Embarrassed by this, the sailor refers to yet another cliché of Soviet media that they "are spilling blood now."[30] Katia asks him if he ever felt remorse or self-loathing for murdering so many people, which he prefers not to answer. She interrupts his monologue about the beauty of collective labor with a rhetorical question, asking if they would not like to get back to peaceful work in the fields on their land. Suddenly, the sailor's friend (who was also a former peasant) agrees that it would be nice to live as people did in the old good times under Nicholas II. Then the conversation terminates, and the reader can interpret the silence as a discrepancy between what people are forced to think and what they secretly feel. Veresaev shows quite prophetically that ideology, although playing a significant role in pushing citizens to behave violently, is not something they completely agree with. Individuals, regardless of which side they defend, strive for peace.

Nevertheless, Veresaev demonstrates how the propaganda of extermination affects people's behavior as a viral infection. A good example to illustrate this point is the story of Professor Dmitrevskii and the Bolshevik newspaper. Professor Dmitrevskii, who sided with the Bolsheviks and started working for a public education center, gives a public talk. In the end, he enthusiastically exclaims that science and education for the working class are more efficient than using a gun. The local reporter writes an article in which he distorts the professor's final thought and says quite the opposite: socialism should be built only with force and violence: "by a worker holding a rifle and a bayonet in his calloused hand."[31] Despite the professor's pleas, the editorial board did not correct the quote. The editorial tactics here bear a resemblance to the central argument in Elaine Scarry's book *The Body in Pain*, where she examines the connection between violence and the language of war. Scarry highlights its misuse, how it omits and re-describes physical injuries, making them invisible for the war participants.[32] Veresaev marks the belligerent rhetoric of the Bolsheviks who appear to follow the same pattern: they depersonalize human beings, avoiding mentioning their physical suffering.

Professor Dmitrevskii's words lose their expressivity and peaceful meaning, once the journalist transforms them into a distorted message, that has another purpose: to instigate class struggle.

The effect of the propagandistic rhetoric is precisely the reason why a peaceful talk cannot prevent violence. The Reds arrest landowners, mostly the elderly, and send them to dig trenches. Katia's father, Doctor Sartanov, defends the sick priest Vosdvizhenskii and tries to convince Khanov to release him; otherwise, Vosdvizhenskii will not survive the journey. The perpetrator refuses to listen to the doctor's arguments, and the priest dies in a basement. The journey results in sending the arrested back because the commandant did not need, using his own words, "that rubbish."[33] Human beings are treated as things, and the death of an individual looks like a byproduct of the new bureaucracy. The doctor's words do not stop an agent of violence from locking a sick man in a basement. In the words of Giorgio Agamben from his well-known essay "On the Limits of Violence" (1970), Veresaev shows that language as "the power we wield against death" is separated from violence.[34]

In one of the fiercest disputes between Katia and her cousin Leonid (a proponent of Bolshevism) Katia accuses the Bolsheviks of murdering people without trial and mistreating prisoners, something unimaginable in Imperial Russia. Leonid disagrees and says that the new social order requires violent measures to eliminate opposition. One side is terrified to see themselves as an accidental victim as much as the other is excited to be a vengeful perpetrator. One side is eager to continue the conversation, hoping that the other agrees to make peace, whereas the latter wants to interrupt communication—Leonid says that "we are not going to show any deference to the bourgeoise."[35] The exchange ends in silence, which signifies intransigence on both ends.

One may wonder why dialogues flow so naturally and peacefully even if the characters do not reach an amicable agreement. One of the most original features of Veresaev's literary work is that his main character is the beautiful young girl, Katia. In fairness, we should note that several of Veresaev's other novels and stories also feature women as main protagonists, such as Natasha in *Impassability* (1894), Varvara Vasilievna in *On the Curve* (1901), and Lel'ka and Ninka in the novel *Sisters* (1933).[36] Katia's young age combined with her predisposition for empathetic listening and sincerity allow her to safely enter discussions with both sexes. She represents Veresaev's healthiest human personality, which means a non-violent person. The author describes Katia's conversational behavior as a childish, naïve, and impulsive reaction to someone else's words. And hence one may discover another distinct feature of the narrative, the uncanonical representation of Soviet femininity. While historians of Soviet gender such as Choi Chatterjee and Elizabeth Wood point to the New Soviet Woman which served as "the embodiment of Soviet belief in gender equality"[37] and played the most important role in the war that "was to influence their husbands, brothers, and sons to go off to fight and not shirk their responsibilities,"[38] Veresaev created his own ideal image of a woman, contradicting the officially propagated militarized portrait. As a matter of fact, such a representation of emphasized femininity is found in the traditional depiction of Red Cross nurses in Imperial Russia. Susan Grant in her article "Nurses in the Soviet Union: Explorations of Gender in State and Society" argues that "prior to the Bolshevik takeover of power in October 1917, the nursing profession was similar to nursing in other countries in that it was based on Christian values and a religious ethos."[39] Though one could call Katia a nurse only metaphorically, she treats people gently, demonstrating kindness and care, patiently listening to their complaints, accusations, and even "belligerent rhetoric." The role of empathetic listener more appropriately fits the image of a doctor or nurse in Pre-Revolutionary Russia than it does the new Soviet canonization of women, who were viewed as "no less active agents of revolution or counterrevolution than were men."[40] Katia cannot come to terms with her sister or Uliasha, who conversely show that they are "worthy of this great revolution" in which they are "participants," to borrow Grigorii Zinoviev's[41] words on the pivotal role the "baba" or woman plays in the struggle for liberation, from his speech at the 1919 Petrograd Second City Conference for Women Workers.[42]

At the same time, Veresaev's choice of a female heroine, taking into consideration how much attention the Soviet state paid to establishing new gender regulations aimed toward equality between women and men, could be a strategy to withstand the pressures of censorship. Women assumed the caring and nurturing roles within Soviet society,[43] and the censor was very likely to see in Katia the transitional type of a protagonist who must eventually transform herself into the epitome of a Soviet "baba" revolutionary.

However, Katia is so alone in her search for humanism and therefore so likely to be exposed to the fast-spreading epidemic of violence that she seems *to get sick*, shooting a Ukrainian anarchist to save her cousin's life and feeling excited about it. Nevertheless, the writer endeavors *to treat* his favorite protagonist. In the same chapter, Katia runs into the most dangerous and cruel executioner, Voron'ko. Initially, she doesn't know who he is and likes his confident manner of speaking and intelligent appearance. Presumably, Voron'ko's prototype is Dzerzhinsky, the director of the Soviet Secret Police, mentioned above. Under his guidance, thousands of political opponents were shot without trial in the basements of prisons and public places. Katia tries to read his face for signs of guilt (she calls it "world sadness," a formulation that could reference the Byronic romantic hero), or pathology (resembling Dostoevsky's terrorists from *Demons*) and instead is terrified to see that he looks like a healthy, intelligent man with strong opinions. She asks him if it was necessary to execute the innocent, and he defends his position by advocating for terror. He openly says that the untraceable disappearance of people in basements without public executions and final statements from the convicted offenders are needed to find the internal enemy. It is better to murder ten innocent people than miss one worthy of blame. Katia is horrified and doubts his words, attributing them to theoretical speculation until she learns his name. The conversation stops and confuses her because she cannot reconcile his friendly countenance and family role as a father with his identity as an executioner. Violence is normalized, and this is something Katia cannot accept. In this she strongly resembles Veresaev himself, who takes a humanitarian, Hippocratic approach to both patient and character alike.

Thus far I have paid considerable attention to conversations in the narrative to demonstrate the diagnostic nature of the communication between the main protagonist (Katia, a doctor) and her interlocutors (patients). However, we could also analyze the authorship and narrative structure of *The Deadlock* from the perspective of therapeutic writing. In the novel, dialogues are written from the perspective of multiple voices which do not move the action or the relationship forward. Veresaev needs the presence of the Other to create the kind of mental activity that resists violence and the external pressures of totalitarianism. In this sense, his novel may be interpreted using both Hannah Arendt and Mikhail Bakhtin's view on Socrates' dialogues which strangely overlap in Veresaev's case. Hannah Arendt in her book *The Life of the Mind* poses the following ethical question: "Could the activity of thinking as such, the habit of examining whatever happens to come to pass or to attract attention, regardless of results and specific content, could this activity be among the conditions that make men abstain from evil-doing?"[44] She refers to Socrates as a thinking subject, claiming that in times of the abolition of human rights and morality, the ability to question new norms keeps individual identity safe from the detrimental effects of ideology. Similarly, Bakhtin juxtaposes the Socratic dialogues to an official monologism that possesses absolute truth. Julia Kristeva, who was among the first to introduce Bakhtin's work to a Western audience, in her pivotal essay "Bakhtin, Word, Dialogue and Novel," points to the exceptional situation of the threshold of death, in which Socrates makes his speech of legal self-defense at the trial in Plato's *Apology*. She emphasizes that, for Bakhtin, the speaker's agency loses its representational function, giving way to symbolic meanings when "speech, commensurating with the speech of the other, comes in touch with death."[45] And, resonating with Arendt and Bakhtin, in the proximity of death in the Civil War, Veresaev saturates his story with conversations that, on one hand, seem to save the self from the epidemic of violence, and, on the other, de-subjectivizes speech that becomes actualized only when it concerns others, only via the author's empathetic understanding of the Other in a communicative act. One may conclude that, although in the novel the spoken word does not prevent harm, for Veresaev, the possibility of an open discussion, verbalized in a narrative, becomes a therapeutic process of writing.[46]

One should consider which events of the Civil War Veresaev reconstructs. To my mind, the way Veresaev selects those situations can be compared with how a physician assesses the general health of a person and concludes that the patient has severe health problems. He shows moments which Foucault called "microphysics of power."[47] Veresaev describes in detail the arrests of landowners, Katia's imprisonment, her father's staged execution, and the heroic death of Katia's sister Vera in a mass shooting by White officers. Each situation manifests itself as abnormal. The landowners are shown as old, sick, poor, and unarmed. They do not look like backstabbing enemies of the Revolution but, nevertheless, they are treated as such and arrested. Katia wants to make her own decision about with whom to share a room and rebukes the accommodation manager for his obtrusive manners. Katia is arrested because she told the property manager that this "Kingdom of Ham" should end one day. These words were immediately interpreted as counter-revolutionary, which results in accusations of treason and even a death sentence. When talking to her cousin, Katia compares conditions for prisoners in the Tsarist times, when they were treated with respect, allowed to get some fresh air, and given enough food, and under the Bolsheviks, who treat people like cattle and keep them in icy cold cellars. Her father is released but has to experience a mock execution from which he cannot mentally recover and soon thereafter dies. The Whites arrest Katia's sister Vera, and as if the death sentence did not seem enough, they put her in a cell with male prisoners the night before the execution. The violence Veresaev describes has no ideological grounds and demonstrates pathological forms of power.

One might want to emphasize the scene of Vera's heroic acceptance of her impending death at the shooting site. Veresaev shows her as a genuine believer in her sacrifice, which is needed to build a Brave New World and which future generations will remember as her ultimate act of heroism. And here again, it may be fruitful to refer to Agamben who argued that "revolutionary violence can be described as passion, in its etymological sense: self-negation and self-sacrifice. When seen from this perspective, it becomes clear that repressive violence (which enforces law) and delinquent violence (which defies law) are no different from the violence aimed at establishing new laws and new power: in each case, negation of the other fails to become negation of the self."[48] All the Bolsheviks are shown as passionate believers ready to sacrifice human lives for building a new world. One may say that they *self-negate* when they carry out executions of their own members (in the novel, a property manager was killed by Voron'ko for corruption) and *self-sacrifice* when they accept being executed by the opposite party (Vera's shooting as an act of self-sacrifice).

Vikentii Veresaev is a careful examiner of the Russian Revolution and the Civil War. His doctor's eye notices the situations which intellectuals of the second half of the twentieth century up to the present day continue to discuss extensively: structured violence, mass shootings in the totalitarian state, the normalization of violence, and the propaganda of extermination. His diagnostic approach detects how ideology propagates aggression toward the educated class and how supporters of the Bolsheviks and the White movement both use their political preferences as an excuse to exercise power. He also attempts to convert violence into an open peaceful conversation; however, most of them end in a deadlock.

Veresaev depicts violence as an epidemic that his characters cannot escape. The disease turns out to be incurable, though therapeutic communication may relieve some symptoms. However, none of the protagonists can avoid becoming either a victim or a perpetrator in the harsh reality of the Civil War. Katia's disappearance in the end shows the author's confusion. In his last novel *Sisters*, written in the 1930s, Veresaev would make another attempt to fit his main protagonists, young women Lel'ka and Ninka, into the new Soviet society, while his novel about life at a shoe factory, *The Red Bogatyr*, resembles the first narratives of Socialist Realism. Veresaev did intend to create a text relevant to workers and accessible to them, but also aspired to orient himself in the new Soviet cultural environment.[49] Unlike Ninka and Lel'ka, who were able to chart their own path of integration into the new Soviet community, Veresaev did not become a Soviet ideological writer. When *Sisters* came out in 1933, it was severely criticized. Unsurprisingly, during the time of Stalin's Great Purges, Veresaev tried to distance himself from legalized violence. His internal emigration resulted in preparing translations from Homer and Hesiod, writing memoirs and literary criticism.[50]

NOTES

1. The novel's original Russian title is *V tupike*.
2. Veresaev, Vikenty, *Vospominaniia,* Moscow: Pravda, 1982, 335–336.
3. For a more detailed analysis of the stages of medical professionalization in Russia, see Bogdanov, Konstantin, *Vrachi, patsienty, chitateli,* Moscow: Azbuka, 2005.
4. It is necessary to point out the state's Janus-faced attitude to medicine and science. According to the historian Alexander Vucinich, "the tsarist government's decidedly ambivalent attitude toward science, which was best expressed in its

educational policies. On the one hand, the government saw science as indispensable to the modernization of Russia's economy, armed forces, and public services; on the other, it distrusted the scientific spirit, with its critical attitude toward authority, its relativistic interpretation of nature and social institutions, its individualistic approach to problems, and its belief in the supreme wisdom of man's rational capacities" (Introduction, *Science in Russian Culture,* Stanford, Calif.: Stanford University Press, 1963, xi).

5. For an illustrative example of such collaboration, see Charlotte Henze's study *Disease, Health Care and Government in Late Imperial Russia: Life and Death on the Volga, 1823–1914*, Abingdon & New York: Routledge, 2011, in which she examines the history of a cholera epidemic in the Russian town of Saratov.

6. During the last two decades of the nineteenth century, *Vrach* laid the foundation of professional ethics for the medical field in Russia. The brief sketch of the medical community that I have provided is based on archival research I did in the summer of 2019 at the National Library of Medicine, where the whole run of the journal's twenty-two annual volumes is available on microfilm.

7. Lermontov, Mikhail, "Predislovie," *Geroi nashego vremeni*, *Polnoe sobranie sochinenii*, Moscow: Academia, 1937, 186. The original quote is "Budet i togo, chto bolezn' ukazana, a kak ee izlechit'—eto uzh bog znaet!"

8. Critical realism was a disputed but nonetheless commonly used literary term in the 1920s, as well as in Soviet scholarship. For an overview of the application of the term in Russian scholarship of the 1920s and its relation to writer Nikolai Gogol, see V.Vinogradov's article "Gogol i naturalnaia shkola" (1925).

9. For more on the radicalization of the Russian intelligentsia, see Mogilner, Marina, *Mifologiia "podpol'nogo cheloveka": radikal'nyi mikrokosm v Rossii nachala XX veka kak predmet semioticheskogo analiza*, Moscow: Novoe literaturnoe obozrenie, 1999.

10. The Russian for this term is "Podpolnaya Rossiia."

11. For more on the history of the Pirogov Congresses, especially the 1905 Pirogov Congress, where the members all agreed that the political system needs to be reformed, see, for example, Frieden, Nancy, *Russian Physicians in an Era of Reform and Revolution, 1856–1905*, Princeton, New Jersey: Princeton University Press, 2014, Appendix V.

12. The original Russian title of this work is *Zapiski vracha*. As Veresaev says in his diary of 1945, "The medical press gave my book a hostile reception" [translation mine].

13. The original Russian is "zhizn' grubaia, gromadnaya i moguchaia."

14. For more on Veresaev's life and works, see Brovman, G. E., *Veresaev. Zhizn' i tvorchestvo,* Moscow: Sovetskii pisatel, 1959, and Nolde, Valeriia, *V.M. Veresaev–zhizn' i tvorchestvo*, Tula: Priokskoe knizh. izd-vo, 1986.

15. In Ivan Bunin's *The Cursed Days* the narrator lists multiple examples of the Bolsheviks' crimes, calling Soviet reality "The Kingdom of Ham." Alexey Remizov concludes in his *Slovo o pogibeli russkoi zemli* (1917) that all saints left Russia at the darkest hour of the Revolution; Isaac Babel in *The Red Cavalry* (1926) transforms battle scenes into a mythological space where natural landscapes and even church

bells speak the language of violence; Boris Pilnyak alludes to the evil spirits (*nechist'*) of Russian folklore and depicts the new world as barbaric in *The Naked Year* (1922); at the other end of the symbolic spectrum is Dmitrii Furmanov who creates an adventure story about the people's hero *Chapaev* (1923).

16. The original Russian for the process is "likvidatsiiu izlishkov u burgiuazii."

17. Veresaev, Vikenty, *V tupike*, *Sestry*, Moscow: Knijnaia palata, 1990, 185.

18. The novel came out in 1923.

19. Chamberlin, William Henry, "The Tragedy of the Russian Intelligentsia," *The Russian Review* 18. 2 (1959): 94.

20. For more on "humanitarian narratives," see Laqueur, Thomas, "Bodies, Details, and the Humanitarian Narrative," *The New Cultural History*. Eds. Biersack, Aletta. Berkeley: University of California Press, 1989.

21. Laqueur, *Bodies, Details, and the Humanitarian Narrative,* 201.

22. Kleimann, Arthur, *The Illness Narratives*, New York: Basic Books, 1988, 27.

23. Kleimann, *The Illness Narratives*, 11.

24. Translation mine. The original quote is "sovokupnuiu zhisn' bol'nogo organisma vo vsekh otlichiiakh ot zdorovogo," Veresaev, Vikenty, *Zapiski vracha*. http://az.lib.ru/w/weresaew_w_w/text_0030.shtml. Accessed November 20, 2018. No pagination.

25. The original title of the miscellany is *Bolnaya Rossiia.* See the original quote in Merezhkovskii's article about Boris Savenkov's novel *The Pale Horse* (*Kon' Bledny*) (1909): "Zakonnoe nasilie dlya nas pochti neoschiutimo, potomu shto slishkom privychno [. . .] eto ezhesekundnoe krovoprolitie tak zhe besboleznenno, kak pravilnoe dvizheniie krovi v zhilakh." Merezhkovskii, Dmitrii, "Kon' Bledny," *Bolnaya Rossiia.* http://az.lib.ru/m/merezhkowskij_d_s/text_1909_kon_bledny.shtml. Accessed December 2, 2019. No pagination.

26. A fruitful point of comparison to Veresaev's work is Mikhail Bulgakov's story collection *A Country Doctor's Notebook*, which is analyzed further in the present volume in the chapters by Miller. Like Veresaev, Bulgakov received a medical education and later became a writer. The stories were published in 1925–1927, and one may examine how Bulgakov situates his main protagonists in the Civil War. Two stories, directly referring to this period, are quite different. The story "I Killed" is about Doctor Yashvin, who violates medical ethics when he kills colonel Leschenko, a war criminal, on the operating table. Another story, "Morphine," contains an episode about a doctor who became a morphine addict and during the Civil War escaped from a Moscow hospital, taking advantage of the revolutionary chaos and stealing drugs from pharmacies. Both examples feature a surgeon who is either infected with the surrounding violence and becomes a killer himself or self-destructs, developing a drug addiction to escape from reality. Both examples demonstrate that Bulgakov's stories cannot be named diagnostic narratives.

27. The English translation from Veresaev's *V tupike* will be quoted from Nina Wissotzky and Camilla Coventry's *The Deadlock* unless otherwise noted. This quotation is found on page 50. Russian quotations from Veresaev's *V tupike. Sestry* will also be provided when necessary.

28. Bunin, Ivan, *Dnevnik 1917–1918*, vol. 8, Moscow: Moskovsky rabochy, 2000, 60.

29. The original Russian for this term is "kafedra bezbozhiia" (Lebina, Natalia, *Sovetskaia povsednevnost': Normy i anomalii. Ot voennogo kommunisma k bolshomu stiliu*, Moscow: Novoe literaturnoe obozrenie, 2015, 197).

30. Veresaev, *V tupike*, 81. The original Russian is "my seichas krov' prolivaem" (translation mine).

31. Veresaev, *V tupike,* 99. The original Russian is "tolko besposchadnoi vintovkoi i shtykom v mozolistoi ruke rabochego" (translation mine).

32. See Scarry, Elaine, "The Structure of War: The Juxtaposition of Injured Bodies and Unanchored Issues," *The Body in Pain. The Making and Unmaking of the World*, New York, Oxford: Oxford University Press, 1985.

33. Veresaev, *The Deadlock*, 140.

34. Agamben, Giorgio, "On the Limits of Violence." Eds. Lorenzo Fabbri, trans. Elizabeth Fay. *Diacritics* 39.4 (2009): 109. I should clarify though that for Agamben language is the only possible space for reconciliation, while for Veresaev in most cases it is not.

35. Veresaev, *V tupike,* 41. The original Russian is "A burzhuasiia, - da, s neiu tseremonitsa my ne stanem" (translation mine).

36. The original Russian titles of these novels are *Bez dorogi*, *Na povorot'e*, and *Sestry*, respectively.

37. Chatterjee, Choi, "The Public Identity of Soviet Women," *Celebrating Women. Gender, Festival Culture, and Bolshevik Ideology, 1910–1939*, Pittsburgh, PA: University of Pittsburgh Press, 2002, 138–139.

38. Wood, Elizabeth A., *The Baba and the Comrade: Gender and Politics in Revolutionary Russia*, Bloomington: Indiana University Press, 1997. 59.

39. Grant, Susan, "Nurses in the Soviet Union: Explorations of Gender in State and Society," *Women and Gender in Twentieth-Century Russia and the Soviet Union*, Eds. Melanie Ilic, London: Palgrave Macmillan, 2018, 250.

40. Grant, "Nurses in the Soviet Union," 254.

41. Grigorii Zinoviev was a Soviet Communist politician and one of the seven members of the first Politburo. He was also a proponent of socialist militarism and one of the most powerful leaders during Lenin's final illness in 1922–23.

42. Wood, *The Baba and the Comrade,* 60.

43. Wood, *The Baba and the Comrade,* 60.

44. Arendt, Hannah, *The Life of the Mind*, New York: Harvest Book, 1978, Vol. I, 5.

45. Kristeva, Julia, "Bakhtin, Slovo, Dialogue i Roman," *Frantsuskaia semiotika: Ot strukturalisma k poststructuralismu.* Eds. Kosikov, Georgii, Moscow: Progress, 2000, 427–457. The translation here is mine.

46. It is interesting that Bakhtin's early works, which manifest his developing, not yet dialogical line of thinking and discover the presence of the Other and the importance of the Other to constitute the image of the self, were written in 1919–1924, around the same time Veresaev completed his novel. For more about communication as an existential strategy see Clark C., Kholkvist M., "Arkhitektonika otvetstven-

nosti," *Mikhail Bakhtin: pro et contra,* St. Petersburg: Russkii Christianskii gumanitarny institut, 2002, 59.

47. Foucault, Michel, *Discipline and Punish–The Birth of the Prison*. Trans. Alan Sheridan. New York: Vintage Books, 1995, 28.

48. Agamben, "On the Limits of Violence," 108.

49. The writer feared being alienated from the proletariat, much like his main protagonists. The main characters in *Sisters* create a diary, a narrative project, that allows them to develop strategies for navigating the uncanny spaces of everyday life and re-establish their sense of place. In their diary, they reproach themselves for excessive sensitivity and label it as a class-marked deficiency. They abandon their sentimentality and femininity because they associate them with the decadent aristocracy that prevents them from becoming Soviet citizens. However, the novel ends tragically. A secondary character Yurka, Lel'ka's former boyfriend, hangs himself because he cannot forgive himself for the violence he committed against a little boy, whose last pair of winter boots he took away during a dekulakization raid. The epidemic of violence kills him.

50. In "The Tragedy of the Russian Intelligentsia" Chamberlin comes exactly to the same conclusion, saying that "when the pressure of ideological conformity became extreme, Veresaev stopped writing on current themes and prepared some scholarly works on Pushkin and some translations of classical Greek poems. It was in this kind of 'internal emigration' that many of the old Russian intelligentsia remained intellectually active and at peace with their consciences," 94.

WORKS CITED

Agamben, Giorgio. "On the Limits of Violence." Eds. Lorenzo Fabbri, trans. Elizabeth Fay. *Diacritics* 39.4 (2009): 103–111.

Arendt, Hannah. *The Life of the Mind*. New York: Harvest Book, 1978, Vol. I.

Babel, Isaak. *Konarmiia*. Moscow: Vremya, 2017.

Bogdanov, Konstantin. *Vrachi, patsienty, chitateli*. Moscow: Azbuka, 2005.

Brovman, G.E. *Veresaev. Zhizn' i tvorchestvo*. Moscow: Sovetskii pisatel, 1959.

Bulgakov, Mikhail. "Morphii." *Izbrannoe*. Moscow: Khudozhestvennaia literatura, 1980. 346–370.

Bulgakov, Mikhail. "Ya ubil." *Izbrannoe*. Moscow: Khudozhestvennaia literatura, 1980. 374–383.

Bunin, Ivan. *Dnevnik 1917–1918*, vol. 8. Moscow: Moskovsky rabochy, 2000.

Bunin, Ivan. *Okayannye dni*. Saint Petersburg: Azbuka, 2014.

Chamberlin, William Henry. "The Tragedy of the Russian Intelligentsia." *The Russian Review* 18.2 (1959): 89–95.

Chatterjee, Choi. "The Public Identity of Soviet Women." *Celebrating Women. Gender, Festival Culture, and Bolshevik Ideology, 1910–1939*. Pittsburgh, PA: University of Pittsburgh Press, 2002.

Clark C., Kholkvist M. "Arkhitektonika otvetstvennosti." *Mikhail Bakhtin: pro et contra.* Saint Petersburg: Russkii Christianskii gumanitarny institut, 2002.

Fokht-Babushkin, Iu.U. "Vikenty Veresaev." *Russkaia literatura rubezha vekov (1890–nachalo 1920 godov)*. Eds. V.A. Keldush. Kniga 1. Moscow: RAN, 2001.
Fokht-Babushkin, Iu.U. "V.V. Veresaev–Leghendy i realnost." *Veresaev V.V., sochinenii v chetyrekh tomakh.* Vol.1. Moscow: Pravda, 1990.
Furmanov, Dmitrii. *Chapaev*. Moscow: Eksmo, 2013.
Foucault, Michel. *Discipline and Punish–The Birth of the Prison*. Trans. Alan Sheridan. New York: Vintage Books, 1995.
Frieden, Nancy. *Russian Physicians in an Era of Reform and Revolution, 1856–1905*. Princeton, New Jersey: Princeton University Press, 2014.
Grant, Susan. "Nurses in the Soviet Union: Explorations of Gender in State and Society." *Women and Gender in Twentieth-Century Russia and the Soviet Union*, Eds. Melanie Ilic. London: Palgrave Macmillan, 2018.
Henze, Charlotte. *Disease, Health Care and Government in Late Imperial Russia: Life and Death on the Volga, 1823–1914*. Abingdon & New York: Routledge, 2011.
Kleimann, Arthur. *The Illness Narratives*. New York: Basic Books, 1988.
Kristeva, Julia. "Bakhtin, Slovo, Dialogue i Roman." *Frantsuskaia semiotika: Ot strukturalisma k poststructuralismu.* Eds. Kosikov, Georgii. Moscow: Progress, 2000. 427–457.
Laqueur, Thomas. "Bodies, Details, and the Humanitarian Narrative." *The New Cultural History*. Eds. Biersack, Aletta. Berkeley: University of California Press, 1989.
Lebina, Natalia. *Sovetskaia povsednevnost': Normy i anomalii. Ot voennogo kommunisma k bolshomu stiliu*. Moscow: Novoe literaturnoe obozrenie, 2015.
Lermontov, Mikhail. *Geroi nashego vremeni.* In Volume V of his *Polnoe sobranie sochinenii*. Moscow: Academia, 1937. 185–321.
Merezhkovskii, Dmitrii. "Kon' Bledny." *Bolnaya Rossiia*. http://az.lib.ru/m/merezhkowskij_d_s/text_1909_kon_bledny.shtml. Accessed December 2, 2019. No pagination.
Mogil'ner, Marina. *Mifologiia "podpol'nogo cheloveka": radikal'nyi mikrokosm v Rossii nachala XX veka kak predmet semioticheskogo analiza*. Moscow: Novoe literaturnoe obozrenie, 1999.
Nolde, Valeriia. *V.M. Veresaev–zhizn' i tvorchestvo*. Tula: Priokskoe knizh. izd-vo, 1986.
Pilnyak, Boris. *Goly god. Povest' nepogashennoi luny. Rasskazy.* Moscow: AST, 2009.
Remizov, Alexey. *Slovo o pogibeli russkoi zemli.* https://rvb.ru/remizov/ss10/tocvol_5.htm. Accessed June 5, 2019.
Scarry, Elaine. "The Structure of War: The Juxtaposition of Injured Bodies and Unanchored Issues." *The Body in Pain. The Making and Unmaking of the World.* New York, Oxford: Oxford University Press, 1985.
Veresaev, Vikenty. *Vospominaniia*. Moscow: Pravda, 1982.
Veresaev, Vikenty. *V tupike. Sestry*. Moscow: Knijnaia palata, 1990.
Veresaev, Vikenty. *Zapisi dlya sebya*. http://az.lib.ru/w/weresaew_w_w/text_1945_zapisi_dlya_sebya.shtml. Accessed November 23, 2019. No pagination.

Veresaev, Vikenty. *Zapiski vracha*. http://az.lib.ru/w/weresaew_w_w/text_0030.shtml. Accessed November, 20 2018. No pagination.

Veresaev, V V. *The Deadlock*. Trans. Nina Wissotzky and Camilla Coventry. Westport, Conn.: Hyperion Press, 1973.

Vinogradov, Viktor. *Gogol i naturalnaya shkola*. Leningrad: Obrazovanie, 1925.

Vucinich, Alexander. *Science in Russian Culture*. Stanford, Calif.: Stanford University Press, 1963.

Wood, Elizabeth A. *The Baba and the Comrade: Gender and Politics in Revolutionary Russia*. Bloomington: Indiana University Press, 1997.

Chapter Eight

Wards of the State

Russian Medical Fiction

Angela Brintlinger

For well over a century, Russian writers have used their literary works to confront problems within the medical establishment. Underqualified and underequipped medical personnel, uncaring or ineffective treatment of patients, problematic conditions not conducive to health and healing: fiction has been a place to depict medical situations and to describe their inadequacy. However, throughout this long history of literary lamentations over the state of medical care in Russia, and in the Soviet Union and its successor states, fiction has also been used to indict the political and social conditions that permit the status quo, and authors have clearly identified the medical woes of their country with the larger problems of Russian society. In that sense, the medical ward has frequently been used as a microcosm of Russia itself.

Scholars have explored the literary representation of psychiatric hospitals and care in Russia and the Soviet Union and have made the connections between a mad society and its lunatic inmates.[1] The present chapter will explore the one hundred plus year phenomenon of using not merely psychiatric, but medical space more generally, for the purpose of social commentary. Medical narratives—in various genres, from short story to lengthy novel—explore the power dynamic inherent in the doctor-patient relationship and how that dynamic plays out in medical space, with patients subordinated to the not always competent medical authorities. Further, these fictional texts offer two levels of authority—on one hand, the medical personnel who have knowledge and power over their subordinated patients, and on the other hand the authors of texts who manipulate descriptions, plot, and characters to depict and indict the conditions of medical settings of all kinds and indeed of medical personnel. Authors who have been educated and even worked as doctors find material in their own practices as well as in the medical milieux they witness, and patients subjected to medical procedures and care repurpose their experiences in fictional renditions. In the end, these texts comment on medicine, but more pointedly on larger structures of political authority, using the medical ward as a microcosm and the power dynamic of doctor-patient as a stand-in for the leader-people dynamic.

This essay will take medical texts or sets of texts—authored by four Russian writers—from across the Russian, Soviet, and post-Soviet literary landscape to argue that the ward is an ideal place to examine these power dynamics. An isolated physical location, a medical ward functions to enable social and political commentary, bringing together patients, and sometimes doctors and medical personnel, and in many cases upending social distinctions (which both highlights the presence of such distinctions in society and renders a certain fantasy justice upon those who thought they were above repercussions and punishment because of their elevated social rank). The space of the medical ward enables conversations and stories that could not take place in a parlor—with its specific social conventions and observed hierarchies—or on a factory floor, where among other things conversations must compete with production and other kinds of work. In the fiction of Anton Chekhov, Alexander Solzhenitsyn, Julia Voznesenskaya, and Maxim Osipov, we see variations in genre, from short story to curated story collection to epic novel, and authority figures—including doctors, scientists, writers, and priests—that together demonstrate a marked continuity in the use of ward spaces across more than 125 years.

HUMANITY AND MEDICAL PRACTICE IN CHEKHOV

Chekhov's story "Ward No. 6" (1892) remains one of the most influential and powerful indictments of the Russian medical system and its practitioners. As Polly Jones has argued, nineteenth-century Russia had a "robust tradition of diagnosing personal and social diseases through literature," and some Soviet literature, too, "hinted at a malady affecting Soviet society," but Anton Chekhov set the standard in Russia for explicitly connecting the hospital and its ward with the world around it.[2]

Chekhov (1860–1904) was a doctor-writer who famously claimed that "medicine is my wife and literature is my mistress."[3] He combined the two in frequently portraying medical situations and highlighting doctors in his stories and plays (as critic Gerald Weales so aptly noted, "doctors are endemic in Chekhov's work").[4] Chekhov's quip about the two "women" in his life underlines the primary concerns of his work: on the one hand he was deeply interested in how to heal humanity, how to identify disease and attempt to alleviate pain, but on the other hand he approached his writing and the social and psychological concerns of the society in which he lived with irony and humor, recognizing that to point out—to diagnose—problems is often the most that a writer, or doctor, can do.

"Ward No. 6" is Chekhov's most prominent and frequently explored medical text, but scholars have looked to other texts as well to understand Chekhov's use of and beliefs about medicine, and this chapter will follow that tradition. In fact, because Chekhov was a student and practitioner of medicine as well as a writer of stories and plays, it is worth exploring his non-fiction to gain a better understanding of his concerns with doctors and medicine. For example, in his private journal Chekhov diagnosed a gendered power dynamic between doctors and their female relatives. To quote from the unpublished journal:

> Conversation during a congress of physicians. First doctor: everything is cured by salt. Second doctor, a military one: everything is cured by not using salt. And both are demonstrating this—one on his wife, the other on his daughter.[5]

The authority of the medical men here—in the professional context of a congress, declaring their sweeping methodologies, arbitrarily describing treatments visited upon their female family members, and casting them as unwitting and/or disempowered patients—is unquestionable, and Chekhov's implicit judgment of his colleagues' arrogance resonates beneath his journal entry. Michael Finke uses this note in his biographical study *Seeing Chekhov* to comment on the confluence of two ideas: Chekhov recognizes the faulty logic and flawed research methodology of doctors who really do not know the etiology of illnesses, and also deliberately points to how these doctors exploit the (powerless) women in their lives as subjects of their medical research. For Finke, the journal entry explains Chekhov's personal aversion to being the subject of the medical gaze, and it highlights Chekhov's ability to ironize about that gaze.

What Chekhov's personal journal also does is to rail against unscientific directions in medical professional practice. Professionalism is a significant concern for Dr. Chekhov and perceiving one's own power and authority is a vital part of ethical professional behavior. In "Ward No. 6," for example, Chekhov's Dr. Ragin wields medical authority without recognizing the damage it can inflict. He only comes to understand its nature from the other side, when he himself is subjected to it as a patient. Dr. Ragin exemplifies the worst impulses of the medical system. And Chekhov knew whereof he wrote. As Doris Vidaver and Maynard Cohen comment, the story "gains a richness of detail from Chekhov's awareness of the most mundane details of hospital life." Specifically, regarding doctors, they list:

> the compulsion to ascend the professional ladder, no matter at whose expense; the consequence of stepping beyond boundaries of objectivity toward the patient; the relentless following of hospital routine to a point of exhaustion, which is peculiar to the medical profession.[6]

Ever sensitive to the value of particulars, Chekhov mines his medical knowledge to bring his reader into the world he is creating. Readers of "Ward No. 6" spend significant amounts of time with Dr. Ragin—in his study as he drinks beer and watches the dust gather on his stacks of medical journals; with his friends as he discusses his philosophy of non-action; and finally in the ward itself where he first sits and talks to the fascinating madman Ivan Gromov and then finds himself, too, relegated to a cot in those dirty, hopeless quarters, once his subordinate turns on him and transforms the powerful doctor into a powerless patient.[7] This mental ward, which to Ragin up until the end was a purely theoretical place of incarceration, becomes a graveyard for his theories and the site of his physical death.

Jones highlights this Chekhov story as an "allegory of the diseases of late imperial society," asserting that "illness literature is rarely just physiological" but often "dramatize[s] personal dramas of morality and spirituality, or allegorize[s] broader crises of social, political, and moral health."[8] For Chekhov, it is all very well and good for medical men to engage in philosophical musing, as Ragin does, but their primary task is to attend to the pain of their patients, something his character Dr. Ragin fails to understand until he himself has lost any power to heal or even alleviate pain in any way. Medical men—at conferences, in their studies—can engage in discussions of treatments, but patients are in the end human beings, and their bodies require action, not merely words and theories. In "Ward No. 6," widely considered to be one of Chekhov's most remarkable stories, Chekhov is questioning whether mental illness can be treated at all, but his turnabout-is-fairplay conclusion demonstrates that an ethical approach requires compassionate treatment of human patients regardless of whether a "cure" can be found. Chekhov here, and elsewhere, elevates the importance of humanity and humane treatment.

In other representations of medical men at about the same time, Chekhov ramps up his irony by moving further away from the practice itself, by leaving the medical ward for the laboratory and in essence removing the patient from the equation. For example, in his 1892 story "The Grasshopper," Chekhov's protagonist is Dr. Dymov's frivolous celebrity-seeking wife, who fails to see her husband's genius until too late.[9] The technical aspects of her physician-husband's job—lab work, patients, autopsies, his scientific writing—interest Olga only as much as they have the potential to interfere with (and alternatively to fund) her own daily life. Her spending beyond their means depends on Dymov's continued good health and ability to perform the job that generates the income to sustain her lifestyle. She seeks to align herself with artists of all kinds—painters, musicians, actors—and longs to be near these talented people, eventually entering into an affair with a painter, and thus demonstrating her preference of the arts over the medical sciences. Dymov tolerates it all and never complains, though the reader senses his humiliation.

Only when the doctor is on his deathbed does his wife long for his gaze to be directed upon her:

> Olga Ivanovna recalled her entire life with him, from beginning to end, in all its detail, and suddenly understood that this was truly an extraordinary, unusual, and, compared to her acquaintances, great man. And remembering how her belated father and all his fellow doctors felt about him, she understood that they had all seen in him a future celebrity.[10]

She calls his name repeatedly, but the passive Dymov has departed this world and can no longer respond. This portrait of Olga Ivanovna gives wives and women a bad name, though the character of the mild, passive workaholic Dr. Dymov is not significantly more positive than the inept Dr. Ragin. Ragin misused his power and misdirected his efforts into philosophizing, and when brought into close contact with an intelligent and interesting patient, he failed to utilize his authority to improve the conditions in the mental ward. Dr. Dymov, on the other hand, moves away from living patients and toward science. He too fails, but he fails differently. The story, in Weales's view, is "too predictably neat in its denouement," and its parodic depiction of the shallow society woman, Olga Ivanovna, might give weight to claims about Chekhov's misogyny. However, her fate is quite similar to that of the hero of "Ward No. 6": like Dr. Ragin, Olga Ivanovna has the tables turned on her. Instead of basking in the glow of her extraordinary husband's medical career, she finds herself the widow of a scientific professional felled by a rookie medical mistake.

These two flawed doctors—one who perishes in a psychiatric ward and the other after a careless error while suctioning diphtheria cells for an experiment—fail to wield their medical authority responsibly, or indeed at all, and differ significantly from the cavalier practitioners detailed in Chekhov's private journal. In other cases, Chekhov's fictional doctors have been more perceptive, able to diagnose the illness of their age, to note the age's lack of clarity and the dearth of appropriate actions available to those who live in it. It was arguably with Chekhov that medical literature in Russia began to serve as specifically social commentary, and Chekhov's observations did not posit change any time soon. In "A Medical Case" (1888), for instance, Dr. Koralyov is dragged from Moscow to an outlying factory one Saturday evening to examine the young heiress to the extensive industrial complex.[11] Both he and the young woman, Liza, understand her problem without naming it aloud: the factory is unclean and unhealthy, the workers are ignorant and exploited, and she stands to benefit from it all. Her troubles are more moral than they are physical, and the doctor's first treatment idea is to distract her. "She should get married as soon as possible," he thinks to himself.[12] But to Liza he instead recites a formula that will become familiar to readers and audiences of Chekhov's plays and stories: "For our children and grandchildren this question, [of] whether they are correct or not, will be decided. They will see more clearly than we have. Life will be good in some fifty years, though it's too bad that we won't be there to see it."[13] This delayed optimism is Chekhov's bromide for the age which scholar Laura Goering has called an age of nervousness.[14]

Dr. Koralyov at least notices his own impotence with his patient, but in "Ward No. 6" four years later Chekhov called this individual responsibility out even more vividly. When Dr. Ragin says, "Wait a bit; when in the distant future, prisons and insane asylums no longer exist, there will be neither bars on the windows nor hospital robes," both his interlocutor, the patient Gromov, and the reader see this as the lazy philosophizing of a man who has the power to improve ward conditions and simply chooses not to bother.[15] On a small scale, Chekhov seems to be arguing, such ineffectiveness and indolence can and should be combatted. But his fiction uses medical environments to comment on society more broadly, and he makes it clear that one energetic Dr. Ragin would not change Russian political structures or social life.

Even doctors who do prescribe treatments are merely artificially dampening the anxieties produced by Russian life. In "Breakdown" (1889), Chekhov's protagonist, the law student Vasiliev, is persuaded by his buddies, a medical student and an art student, to visit the red-light district. Vasiliev has been characterized by a friend as a man with a "talent for *humanity* . . . an ultrasensitive, exquisite sense of pain."[16] The breakdown of the title occurs when Vasiliev recognizes just how miserable the state of prostitution is, and just how powerless women are to escape it. When the friends take Vasiliev to a doctor, the cure for the illness of "humanity" turns out to be drops: morphine and bromide. By dulling his sensitivity to the human condition and in particular to the fate of women in Russian society, Vasiliev is able to carry on. The doctor "perfectly understood both the tears and the despair," and under his treatment Vasiliev's "heart became lighter and lighter, as if it were melting."[17]

Chekhov highlights the power of the (usually male) doctor in his journal entry, condemning the careless non-scientific approach of his medical colleagues, but he also shows the incurable ills Russian society faces in his fictional portrayals of doctors. Frivolous women like Olga Ivanovna in "The Grasshopper" are part of the problem, but the greed, graft, and abuse of power—in psychiatric wards and on factory floors alike, as depicted in "Ward No. 6" and "A Medical Case"—along with limited means to treat society's condition (as presented in "Breakdown") suggest that Chekhov's Russia had a terminal illness that was unlikely to just disappear on its own in fifty, a hundred, or even two hundred years.

LEVELING THROUGH CONFINEMENT AND CARELESSNESS IN SOLZHENITSYN'S *CANCER WARD*

If in Chekhov both writer and doctor wield a certain authority, in the work of Alexander Solzhenitsyn (1918–2008) those roles shift. His novel *Cancer Ward* (written 1966) also conveys human stories through what scholar Susan Smernoff has called the device of "artificial confinement," a device that in this case brings patients and medical personnel together in a cancer hospital in Kazakhstan.[18] Like many of his works, Solzhenitsyn's novel has an autobiographical background: while in exile in Kazakhstan he developed a cancer and was himself treated at a hospital in Tashkent. Thus, as author Solzhenitsyn was drawing on his personal experience as cancer patient. The narrative point of view in his novel empathizes with patients who suffer twice or maybe three times over: at the hands of medical authorities, from the disease itself, and from fellow patients on the ward. Doctors, as in Chekhov, are subject to making errors—in diagnosis, in treatment, and even in medical procedures—but the broader cast of characters in a monumental novel permits tragedy, and irony, to be spread around.

In the Soviet Union, Solzhenitsyn's work circulated only in *samizdat*, no doubt due to his critique of the regime's medical and political structures. Critics have asserted that Solzhenitsyn's goal in using a medical setting in this novel, and particularly the space of the ward, was "to penetrate into the souls and minds of the heroes, to open them before the reader's eyes and to allow an intense and sincere exchange of opinion among them."[19] Wards, barracks, dormitories: these are places where conversations can and do take place as if among equals. We see this kind of sincerity in some of Chekhov's patient Ivan Gromov's statements to Dr. Ragin, but the power differential between the patient and his doctor hinders true communication, and after all, Gromov is considered to be a madman.

The title of Solzhenitsyn's novel has an irony built in: in Russian the word *korpus* refers to a building, often part of a larger complex, and thus *Rakovyi korpus* refers to and has been translated as "Cancer Ward"—that building where the cancer patients are located and where treatment takes place. At the same time, of course, the word corpus is a medical word referring to the body, and the idea of a "cancerous corpus"—a direct translation of the title—hovers in the Russian reader's mind. The hospital ward in Solzhenitsyn's novel features numerous beds filled with sick people from "the most disparate social, cultural, and professional backgrounds."[20] And the cancer patients on the ward are in many cases living out death sentences. As Smernoff points out, both Western and Soviet critics saw *Cancer Ward* as an "explicit condemnation of the cancerous, parasitic growth upon the body of the Russian people—the Stalinist government"—and it is similar in that sense to Chekhov's inherent criticism of tsarist society in his stories.[21] For Solzhenitsyn, the supposed "equal" Soviet society is anything but equal, and his text presents opportunities to highlight that hypocrisy through the words and actions of patients. The ward is a microcosm of society, with all its constituent parts.

Critics of *Cancer Ward* often focus their attention on Oleg Kostoglotov, the former prisoner and exile whose experiences are based on the author's own life, or on Pavel Rusanov, a Communist Party official and Stalinist bureaucrat whose disease has brought him down to the level of those ordinary Soviet citizens whose lives he has made so difficult throughout his career. These are two of the more vivid characters in the novel, and they are placed in direct ideological opposition to each other, among other ways by being treated in the very same hospital ward. In official Soviet rhetoric, *uravnilovka*, or leveling, designates the destruction of class-based access to housing, education, and opportunity. Initially a positive concept in the new Soviet classless society, it became a hated, and ineffective, social policy. Solzhenitsyn does not use the word in his novel, but the concept is there, since he invokes the indiscriminacy of disease that ignores the new Soviet classes. Rusanov's physical and psychological distress vindicates the experiences of Solzhenitsyn's alterego Kostoglotov, who cannot help but feel triumphant at seeing Rusanov brought down too. After all, the Communist Party bureaucrat is one of those responsible for the suffering of millions of Gulag prisoners, including Kostoglotov—if not of course for Kostoglotov's tumor.

Illness is arbitrary, and cancer is perhaps the most arbitrary illness of all. The random and usually inexplicable faulty division of cells that produces cancerous tumors often has no direct cause. Rusanov and his ilk believed that they could protect themselves and create comfortable living conditions by rendering loyal service to the state, but when cancer strikes him, he must confront the fact that as a human being he too is subject to illness, pain, and eventually death. His confinement on a ward with regular Soviet citizens, exiles, and former prisoners of the Gulag system should be his comeuppance, and the threat of death his warning—we are all mortal. The fact that Rusanov remains relatively clueless—firmly convinced that "now he won't die," he is able to deal with having to suffer fate's "humiliation and mockery" in that his bed on the ward positions him "between two exiles."[22] The novel confirms Solzhenitsyn's metaphorical understanding of the Soviet Union as a body ravaged by the cancerous growth of Communism, but the outcome is uncertain. The Rusanovs—like tumors—must be cut out to save the country and its people, though nothing so satisfying actually happens in the course of the novel.

But sometimes there is an identifiable cause for an illness. In the case of Liudmila Dontsova, senior oncologist and head of radiation therapy at the hospital, her many years of dedicated service to patients of all stripes do not save her from the scourge of cancer but indeed doom her to share their fate. Dr. Dontsova becomes patient and victim, developing a cancer of her own due to the fact that Soviet hospitals did not provide radiation medicine workers with the proper protection to use their instruments safely. Daily use of radiation machines on patients resulted in significant exposure to harmful rays for the unprotected practitioners, as well. This is no random act of cell division; the Soviet state and the protocols of its medical practice are directly to blame for her illness. Thus, while Dontsova's cancer tragedy is every woman (and man)'s potential tragedy, it also has a specifically professional aspect.[23] Though it angers her, Dontsova has to come to terms with her illness: "Why does it have to be so unjust?" she asks her old mentor. "Why should I, an oncologist, be struck down by an oncological disease, when I know every single one of them, when I can imagine all the attendant effects, consequences and complications?"[24] Like Marie Curie, whose terminal illness was caused by exposure to radiation, the oncologist succumbs to the radiation treatment she prescribed for others. Metaphorically, in Solzhenitsyn's world those who try to effect cures are not immune to suffering.

These two figures in particular—Rusanov, who deserves to suffer and die for his participation in the Soviet party system, and Dontsova, who works within the medical establishment to heal, and yet suffers anyway—demonstrate the complexity of Solzhenitsyn's novel. Chance leads to retribution against the character who violated human norms and participated in Soviet persecutions for his own private benefit, and pervasive negligence and lack of care for the Soviet caregiver lead to unfair and unjust physical consequences for the cancer doctor. Female (medical) victimhood tempers retribution against (male) political power, and the view from Solzhenitsyn's ward shows both.

WOMEN'S SPACE, WOMEN'S VOICES, WOMEN'S HAPPINESS IN VOZNESENSKAYA'S *WOMEN'S DECAMERON*

Julia Voznesenskaya's *Women's Decameron* (originally published in 1986) is a set of stories narrated by ten women quarantined for ten days in a Soviet maternity ward. These new mothers, looking for a way to pass the time, utilize the framework of Boccaccio's *The Decameron* to create a contemporary, Soviet, ultra-feminized version of that text.[25] The very title of the book brings women squarely into the classical canon: not as objects, but as subjects of narration and narrators themselves, they are handed the metaphorical microphone and given voice. Of course, Voznesenskaya does more than just modify and update *The Decameron*, offering women's stories via women's voices in a Soviet woman's space. With *Women's Decameron* Voznesenskaya joins the Russian national tradition of literary texts addressing medical topics and set in medicalized spaces: the tradition of Chekhov and Solzhenitsyn. Her frame and her female characters follow the tradition by offering social and political critique in a medical setting, but as Linda Hutcheon might say, this is "repetition with . . . difference"—a gender difference.[26]

Voznesenskaya (1940–2015) was an author and a baptized Orthodox Christian, and both of these characteristics placed her in direct opposition to the Soviet state. In conjunction with her creative work, she served a term of forced labor in the mid-60s and in 1976 was sentenced to exile as a dissident who participated in an underground journal. In 1980 she emigrated to Germany with her sons, leaving the Soviet Union for good. Thus, her work, like that of Chekhov and Solzhenitsyn, draws on personal experience and deliberately critiques Russian/Soviet society. Voznesenskaya specifically uses women and women's voices to condemn the social and societal inequalities and divisions among women in the Soviet maternity ward and in society more broadly. The voice of the "author" at the beginning of each chapter and in the heading of each story adds a layer of dissident commentary and an additional ironic voice to the mix, particularly since in using the term *avtor* Voznesenskaya employs the corresponding masculine verb forms, thus underscoring the masculine nature of voices of authority while excluding actual male voices from her narrative entirely. In *Women's Decameron* Voznesenskaya evaluates Soviet society, figuring men as a metaphorical plague, but she also permits her very different female characters to share personal experiences and feelings, to transcend their difference when placed in confinement.

As we have seen above, narrative devices in medical texts often depend on role-playing: Russian writers of medical fiction have combined the roles of historian and diagnostician, of writer and doctor, or indeed of writer and patient who train their gaze on their own doctors, on themselves, and on each other. Choosing to emulate Boccaccio's shared storytelling space, Voznesenskaya does more than simply transform the medieval generic prototype. She posits a female version of the powerful male gaze, flipping the traditional roles between observer and observed that inhere in the doctor-patient relationship so that women patients take charge of determining their own significance.[27] Voznesenskaya's cycle of stories permits women disempowered by their institutionalization in the medical ward to offset a feeling of powerlessness with their own mature voices. By distributing the narratological power, *Women's Decameron* offers a new feminine structure for storytelling that gains its meaning from that very dispersion, from a more grassroots or generalized empowerment. In her book, Voznesenskaya is *everySovietwoman*—through her ten female narrators and the "author" figure, she presents a kind of "dispersed autobiography" of Soviet womanhood. Thus, if Chekhov and Solzhenitsyn's medical stories look at social conditions, finding flaws in doctors, their medical practices and establishments, and the system itself, Voznesenskaya updates quarantine time to celebrate women—and only women—in all their variety.

Originally published in Israel and New York, in both Russian and English, Voznesenskaya's text immediately garnered attention from scholars and general readers outside the Soviet Union. For example, Francine du Plessix Gray—herself a novelist, a feminist, and an astute observer of Soviet life—emphasized the medical, social, and literary contexts of *Women's Decameron*. Voznesenskaya's stories, she argued,

> offer an oblique way of criticizing the scandalously corrupt state of Soviet medicine and other human services [and] the indignities which they particularly inflict on women. But segregated ward settings are also literary ploys which enable literary protagonists to speak with utmost candor and sarcasm on a popular Soviet topic—how to effect the *perestroika* of Russian men. [. . . Finally, such texts] may also mark the nascence, at last, of some form of feminist consciousness.[28]

A women's space gives an opportunity for women's voices to be heard—and they comment on their lives, their opportunities, and their interactions with men. Surprisingly, the pace of quarantine, with its sense of a "time out," does make the Soviet maternity ward in *Women's Decameron* feel somewhat spa-like.[29] No symptoms, and no treatments, get in the way of the conversations. For this reason, Harriet Murav's comparison of this ward to other "place[s] of punitive state control"—army quarters, a prison cell, or the barracks of a concentration camp—seems exaggerated.[30] Clearly a ten-day quarantine due to what is called in the text a "common" skin infection does not a concentration camp make, although Murav's lumping together of such "institutional contexts" reinforces the comparisons made above with male representations of medical experiences, including Chekhov's "Ward No. 6." If Doctor Ragin eventually comes to understand for himself that there is nothing at all general or philosophical about individual physical and psychological suffering, and if in Solzhenitsyn's *Cancer Ward*, it becomes clear that doctors as well as the patients are being poisoned by the treatments they variously prescribe or undergo, and where the very experience of cancer is proposed as an allegory of larger political and social problems, then Voznesenskaya's ward functions to poke fun, seriously, at significant Soviet social concerns. Institutions—like medical wards, orphanages, schools, and army barracks—*are* places of state control, but when quarantine isolates Voznesenskaya's women, the inmates take control of the discourse.[31]

Fascinating storytellers, Voznesenskaya's women narrators fill the maternity ward space with creative individuals. Each woman has her own history and tells numerous stories, some sad, even tragic, but others showing the strength of Soviet women who manage despite difficult historical, social, and personal circumstances. Together they find a way to be gentle with each other and to laugh at their situation. Voznesenskaya strings her stories together with a frame narrative, representing an arch, dissident point of view in the "author's" headings to each chapter, but also gently joking about her own presence. For example:

> The First Day with which it all begins, although it must be said that the majority of books known to us being with the first chapter. Hardly anyone could name a book that began with the last chapter, so that it is not so much this that is significant as the fact that, having agreed to tell each other various stories, the women begin with stories of
> FIRST LOVE.
>
> Once women have made up their minds to divulge their most intimate secrets they will inevitably begin with stories about First Love. So now, after a brief introduction which we also recommend you to read, you will start our book with the first story of First Love.[32]

These stylized, vignette-style introductions to each day add one more voice, the author's voice, which also serves to tie the novel—if we want to call it that—together.

The story opens with Emma, a theater director, who as a serious professional woman has no time to waste. Stuck in quarantine, she tries to "work" and is considering ways she might stage Boccaccio's narrative. In a maternity ward the reader might expect patients to be more focused on what Weldon called the "gentle and endearing passions of motherhood," which the critic asserts with some surprise "seem to be the last thing on their minds."[33] But these women are more than just mothers; they are workers, professionals, sisters, friends, lovers. They are human beings, not merely maternal vessels. Voznesenskaya does not allow motherhood to become their only label, despite their current whereabouts in the maternity hospital.

Voznesenskaya offers an entire slate of individual voices, women who are primarily Russian and/or Jewish, but who present an array of Soviet professions of varying statuses: a few "workers," including Olga, a shipyard worker, Irishka, the secretary of the director of a milk factory, and even Albina, an Aeroflot hostess; several educated professional women: Larisa, who holds a doctorate in biology, Natasha, an engineer, and Emma, the theatre director; and several very specifically Soviet types: Valentina, who is a Party bigwig; Zina, a "woman of no fixed abode"; Galina, a dissident wife; and Nelya, a music teacher who happens to be an Auschwitz survivor. The topics broached in *Women's Decameron* include everything from first love to funny places to have sex to infidelity and jealousy to money, revenge, honorable acts, and luck. The settings span what one critic called "a brilliant spectrum of Soviet daily life in labor camps (where [Voznesenskaya] spent time), country dachas, and urban dormitories."[34] These places, which feature in the stories of the women's past lives, extend the space of the narrative beyond the ward to encompass much of Soviet society, and in the ward the women experience both a respite or break from and also a more intense version of their lives on the "outside," as their stories build on each other and weave the listeners into a community. Women wait, women gossip, women share and emote and suffer, weaving their own narratives, and in the end these women change and change each other, and that too is an effect of Voznesenskaya's tales. Having entered the ward pregnant, they leave no longer pregnant, but through the storytelling experience—the *Decameron* trope—they are transformed in even more significant ways than that.

A dissident author like Voznesenskaya might find that a romantic understanding of respite—as a reprieve from political and psychological haranguing and other difficult conditions experienced in Soviet society—parallels the respite for which many women, especially new mothers, long. The psychological state of a new mother, I would argue, can seem at least as desperate as that of a dissident thinker in a repressive political state—and though it is a temporary condition, it is one that only women are capable of experiencing. Thus, this peculiar chronotope, the maternity ward, can seem difficult to evaluate. Is this "time out" really a respite? is it forced isolation, a kind of imprisonment? The coincidence of the term *confinement*, which once was used to describe women's pregnancy and the process of giving birth, suggests an age-old ambiguity in defining this women's time.

But not only women find that in hospital wards and prison cells, space and time become particularly important. As Joseph Brodsky famously declared:

> Prison is essentially a shortage of space made up for by a surplus of time; to an inmate, both are palpable. Naturally enough, this ratio—echoing man's situation in the universe—is what has made incarceration an integral metaphor of Christian metaphysics as well as practically the midwife of literature. As regards literature, this stands, in a certain sense, to reason, since literature is in the first place a translation of metaphysical truths into any given vernacular.[35]

For Brodsky, time in prison is "palpable"; prison becomes a place of creativity and imprisonment a "midwife" to literature. In *Women's Decameron*, the device of artificial confinement facilitates further gestation and rebirth. Having given birth to new human beings, the women spend their days in quarantine being reborn themselves. If diagnosis is a kind of definition, a way to pigeon-hole and reduce a person to the etiology of a disease, and "diagnosis" in a maternity ward means labeling new mothers as such, acknowledging a medical condition that can forever constrain their identities and social roles, then Voznesenskaya upends these definitions in her ward, allowing her women to be multifaceted and self-contradictory. These are not just new mothers. As a collective, despite or perhaps because of the ways in which they contradict the traditional Soviet definition of acceptable collective identity, they become something more.

In the text of *Women's Decameron* Voznesenskaya asserts hospital space as a timeless space: a space akin to a refuge from plague, but also a place where oral discourse is primary. Other bodily functions, including the "miracle" of birth, are removed from the frame entirely; these women seem to ignore their new maternal status, to find that it fails to define them. The fact that many of these stories are about love, lust, and betrayal in relationships inverts the somatic significance of the setting: though the results of sexual behavior are what brought the women together, it is the behaviors themselves that occupy their thoughts and stories. The sometimes cruel or faceless space of a medical institution is filled with voices, laughter, shared sadness, and relationship-building. Rather than prevention, what we see is cure.

The medical significance of waiting gains further resonance in a Soviet context that required mandatory consumer patience—particularly given line culture, and its concomitant relationships and narratives. From the female perspective, the forty weeks of gestation before the birth of a child represent a specific kind of "time out," an enforced waiting period as a fertilized egg gradually transforms and becomes its own person through birth. But in *Women's Decameron*, waiting becomes its own time-space, a place where language can help offset anxiety, create and undermine hierarchies, and organize value systems. Women's time and the time of patients has no price. It cannot be bought or sold and is sometimes not valued at all. Here, though, time itself takes on a new significance, and women's biographies are made important through their very patience (and indeed their status as patients).

The last stories in *Women's Decameron* are devoted to the concept of luck. The secretary Irishka tells about a woman nicknamed "Lucky Maria," whose luck consisted of a series of disasters—her parents were arrested in the 1930s while she was playing hide-and-seek, and she was saved by her grandmother who visited immediately afterward; she was taken to Siberia by that grandmother just before the war and thus avoided the starvation of the Siege of Leningrad. After Stalin died, she found her exiled parents and was able to provide warm beds for them to die in; she married a good-looking young man who turned out to be a drunk who beat her, but then he ran away with another woman, etc. Finally, she lost her legs in a train accident, and became an invalid, but that too was "lucky," and she figured out that she could go to the hospital every time her money was running low to be treated for alcoholism, and then come back out and drink up the pension that had accumulated. Irishka notes that the maimed alcoholic was "quite a sight to look at, but if a person says she's been fortunate from birth, how can you not believe her?"[36]

In Russian "luck" and "happiness" use the same word. *Schast'e*. Irishka goes on to conclude the novel by claiming that each and every woman on the ward—regardless of how many things went wrong in their lives, despite the sometimes sad or hard luck stories they have spent the ten days sharing—is both happy and lucky. The final words of the novel belong to Larisa, who agrees: while it is true that even in their Soviet life they know how to be happy, "we would like life to be more civilized as well."[37]

HOMAGE TO CHEKHOV IN THE TWENTY-FIRST CENTURY

Part of a larger medical narrative in Russia, one that stems from practitioners of medicine who become writers like Chekhov, and one that sees the ward as a place of confinement, usually in a negative way more similar to a concentration camp or a prison, like Solzhenitsyn, Voznesenskaya's ward stories push against the male medical tradition. For her women characters, being in the hospital is of course about health and recovery, but more important is the culture they co-create as women and the language they find, the *obshchii iazyk* or common tongue, to communicate their life experiences, not just their medical charts. The woman doctor in Solzhenitsyn, and the wives and female patients described in Chekhov, serve to highlight the way in which Voznesenskaya gives women the power to fight their circumstances, to force an optimistic ending under less than ideal circumstances. The fact that in Russian the term for "medical chart" is "*istoriia bolezni*" or "(hi)story of illness" underlines the relationship between illness and etiology and storytelling. Writing your own ending is a luxury that few Russian and Soviet citizens actually had.

The genre of story, of storytelling, is one way Chekhov's influence remains visible throughout the Russian medical canon. Only Solzhenitsyn chooses the unwieldy novel; other authors prefer the episodic, the anecdote, the short story. But it is Chekhov's first play, *The Seagull*, and the fate of its heroine Nina Zarechnaya that inadvertently come to the minds of readers of contemporary Russian short story writer Maxim Osipov, who has recently been fêted as a "new Chekhov"—a true doctor-writer who has not abandoned his first vocation as Chekhov more or less did. "If I had enough ideas, or stamina, to sit and write all day, I might leave medicine behind," he is quoted as saying to journalist Joshua Yaffa.[38] But instead Osipov continues to practice medicine at a hospital in the Central Russian town of Tarusa, and he draws much of his inspiration from the patients he meets there. This location—far from the center, from the railroad, from progress and enlightenment—is only part of what reminds one of Chekhov. Another American reviewer comments, "as we meet the sad, amusing down-on-their-luck contemporary characters, whose physical and emotional ailments and histories are diagnosed with a light touch, who else are we supposed to think of?"[39]

Tarusa, like many places where Chekhov set his plays and stories, is far away from everything. Osipov's fictional rendering of it in his story "Rock, Paper, Scissors" is an isolated place with a "joyless Central Russian sort of beauty." This poignancy, perhaps, this love/hate relationship with one's place of residence, also brings Osipov into close proximity to Chekhov. As Svetlana Alexievich has written, Osipov's prose

> reads like something of a diagnosis: an accurate, unforgiving diagnosis of Russian life. [. . .] Out in the provinces, everything is in full view, more exposed—both human nature and the times beyond the window. [. . .] The author relates to his characters as to patients; he asks them where it hurts.[40]

Like Chekhov, Osipov highlights a provincial actress in another story in the collection *Rock, Paper, Scissors*. Lyubochka is a long-time professional who—like a Nina Zarechnaya reborn in a post-Soviet world—somehow finds herself pregnant. Osipov gives the actress center stage to allow her to describe to her co-worker the vivid and perhaps shocking scene she experiences in an abortion ward. Unlike Voznesenskaya's all-female ward, this one is subjected to incursions by a male voice.

A priest has come to the ward to shame the pregnant girls, and he particularly goes after the actress, accusing her of "wanting the easy life." Actors, he claims, are hypocrites, and "hypocrites will not be saved." Taking the moral high ground, the priest condemns all the pregnant women as sinners who should embrace the suffering their pregnancies imply and bring new life to rebuild post-Soviet society regardless of the details of their sad and complicated lives.

When he finishes his attack on the girls' morals, they explain why they want the abortions in the first place: "I've got no apartment!" "I got laid off!" "Have you seen the waiting lists for kindergarten?" "You don't know what my mother-in-law's like!" The actress, Lyubochka, sums up: "One's unemployed, another has no roof over her head, the third's husband is a drunk."[41] Like Chekhov's patients and provincial dwellers and Voznesenskaya's varied cast of women, the female patients' social conditions help to explain their physical and medical problems. And like his predecessors, Osipov demonstrates that the hospital and the clinic metaphorically stand in for society, a society that in the early twenty-first century is again ailing.

Osipov challenges the religious view that women must fulfill their function as the bearers of children. All the girls, despite the priest's admonitions, go ahead with their abortions, even Lyubochka, who up until then had been undecided about what to do about her pregnancy. If Chekhov's Nina Zarechnaya—a character based in part on his own former love, Lika Mizinova, and her fate as an unwed mother in nineteenth-century Russia—goes through with birthing her child out of wedlock, today's actresses, and other women as well, take a more sensible approach. Practical problems require practical solutions, and despite the girls' wailing, they make the necessary choice. Without the necessary social conditions to bear and raise children, twenty-first-century women try to make their own happiness, to assert their autonomy, in this case by ending their pregnancies.

But every doctor, and every writer, is by necessity a patient as well, and the universality of the experience of patienthood, of being the object of an authoritative voice and gaze, gives a certain flexibility and nuance to the Russian representation of medical scenes (and probably not just Russian). For the most part Russian men who write about medical issues seem to feel compelled to "diagnose" not just their characters, but the society they live in. Voznesenskaya—not trained as a medical professional—uses the setting of the maternity ward to portray another scene, one of mutual communication and understanding, one that validates and highlights women while giving them voice and at least a modicum of agency. In a complex world of disease and disappointment, their conversations and storytelling offer some hope for mutual communication among people of differing status and professions.

Women in these medical stories usually have the role of passive victims, but in Voznesenskaya's writing the women are active, constructing a new world, a real one, not the fake Soviet world that has contributed to their suffering on the outside. *Women's Decameron* highlights that peculiar time-space that blends hospital and prison. It also builds on Russian tradition, exploring notions of time and how time transpires/slows down/engenders creativity and memory. In her novel of many voices, Voznesenskaya also explores notions of women, presented as suppressed wives, passive and sometimes ignorant patients. The outer world of Russian society is sometimes reprised on a micro level in the inner world of the ward, resulting in social commentary and criticism, but in Voznesenskaya in particular it is contrasted to the "safe" or "time out" space of quarantine, where a single-sex conversation enables women to create a female space. Osipov's short stories also give women voice and autonomy, suggesting that medical discourse and authority in fiction cannot necessarily counter the goal of the individual to live a life that is a little more civilized.

NOTES

1. See, for example, Reich, Rebecca, *State of Madness: Psychiatry, Literature, and Dissent After Stalin*, DeKalb: Northern Illinois University Press, 2018. See also Brintlinger, Angela, and Ilya Vinitsky, eds., *Madness and the Mad in Russian Culture*, Ilona Moteiunaite, *Vospriiatie iurodstva russkoi literaturoi XIX–XX vekov*, Toronto: University of Toronto Press, 2007, and Sirotkina, Irina, *Diagnosing Literary Genius: A Cultural History of Psychiatry in Russia, 1880–1930*, Baltimore: Johns Hopkins University Press, 2002.
2. Jones, Polly, "Diagnosing the Stalinist Sickness: Images of Illness in Aleksandr Bek and Aleksandr Solzhenitsyn," *Modern Language Review* 111.4 (October 2016): 1085 and 1090.
3. The Russian versions of Chekhov's letters are from the Academy edition of Chekhov's *Polnoe sobranie pisem v 12 tomakh* (Moscow, 1974–1983). This quotation is from a letter to Alexei Suvorin, Volume II, 326.
4. Weales, Gerald, "Chekhov: The Doctor Is In," *The Sewanee Review* 113, no. 2 (2005): 330.
5. Quoted and discussed in Finke, Michael, *Seeing Chekhov: Life and Art*, Cornell UP, 2005, 57; from Chekhov *Sochineniia* 17: 143. For another view of Chekhov's representation of illness in the context of identity see Popkin, Cathy, "Doctor without Patients/Man without a Spleen: A Meditation on Chekhov's Practice," *Chekhov the Immigrant: Translating a Cultural Icon*. Ed. Michael C. Finke and Julie de Sherbinin. Bloomington, IN: Slavica, 2007.
6. Vidaver, Doris and Maynard M. Cohen, "Vocation: Dr. A. P. Chekhov," *The American Scholar* 55.2 (Spring 1986): 227.
7. Chekhov, "Ward No. 6," in Volume VIII of his Chekhov, Anton, *Polnoe sobranie sochinenii v 18 tomakh*, Moscow: Nauka, 1974–83, 72–126. Hereafter, this collection will be cited as *PSS*, plus the appropriate volume and page numbers.

8. Jones, "Diagnosing the Stalinist Sickness," 1084, 1088.

9. In the Russian, the story is titled "Poprygun'ia."

10. Chekhov, "Poprygun'ia," in *PSS* VIII, pp. 7–31. Quote on p. 30.

11. In the Russian, the story is titled "Sluchai iz praktiki." Chekhov, "Sluchai iz praktiki," in *PSS* X, pp. 75–85.

12. Chekhov, *PSS* X, 78. A woman makes a similar assessment of her best possible future, without the medical context, in Chekhov's "A Woman's Kingdom" (*Bab'e tsarstvo*, 1894).

13. Chekhov, *PSS* X, 85–86.

14. Goering, Laura, "'Russian Nervousness': Neurasthenia and National Identity in Nineteenth Century Russia," *Medical History* 47.1 (2003). See also Morrissey, Susan K., "The Economy of Nerves: Health, Commercial Culture and the Self in Late Imperial Russia," *Slavic Review* 69.3 (Fall 2010).

15. Chekhov, *PSS* VIII, 96.

16. "Breakdown," translated by Jerome Katsell, in *Anton Chekhov's Selected Stories*, 183–201, quote on p. 197. Chekhov, "Pripadok," *PSS* VII, pp. 199–221.

17. Chekhov, "Pripadok," *PSS* VII, 202.

18. Smernoff, Susan S., "The Irony of the Doctor as Patient in Chekhov's 'Ward No. 6' and in Solzhenitsyn's 'Cancer Ward,'" *Chekhov's Art of Writing: A Collection of Critical Essays*. Paul Debreczeny and Thomas Eekman, eds. Columbus, OH: Slavica, 1977, 170.

19. *Cancer Ward* began to circulate in Russian in *samizdat* in 1966, and the novel was finally published in the USSR in 1990. Pervushin, Nikolai V., "Preliminary Remarks on the Literary Craft of Solzhenitsyn," *Canadian Slavonic Papers*, 13.2 & 3 (1971): 141–146, quoted in Smernoff, "The Irony of the Doctor as Patient in Chekhov's 'Ward No. 6' and in Solzhenitsyn's 'Cancer Ward,'" 170.

20. Smernoff, "The Irony of the Doctor as Patient in Chekhov's 'Ward No. 6' and in Solzhenitsyn's 'Cancer Ward,'" 169.

21. Quote in Smernoff "The Irony of the Doctor as Patient in Chekhov's 'Ward No. 6' and in Solzhenitsyn's 'Cancer Ward,'" 170–711. Cf. Rothberg, Abram, *Aleksandr Solzhenitsyn: The Major Novels*, Ithaca: Cornell UP, 1971.

22. Solzhenitsyn, Aleksandr, *Rakovyi korpus,* Paris: YMCA Press, 1970, 316; Solzhenitsyn, Alexander, *Cancer Ward.* Nicholas Bethell and David Burg, trans. New York: The Modern Library, 1995, 376–377. Solzhenitsyn leaves Rusanov's fate unclear, although Dontsova, on her final rounds, predicts that he may not last another year (Russian version 381; English version 458).

23. Smernoff details how some critics have seen Dontsova as an autocrat at the hospital and have compared "medical tyranny" with "political tyranny." See 174–176.

24. Solzhenitsyn, *Rakovyi korpus,* 352; *Cancer Ward*, 422.

25. Of Boccaccio's ten narrators, seven are women. Voznesenskaya may have been fully feminizing the framework of the *Decameron* by making all of hers women, but she also comments on the official Soviet literary doctrine of her time in accessing the Italian author. Boccaccio's collection of tales has been seen as an "epic of the new mercantile individualism" and has also been tied to confessional literature—characteristics that are the polar opposite of declared Soviet values. See Ganim, John M.,

"Chaucer, Boccaccio, Confession and Subjectivity," in *The Decameron and the Canterbury Tales: New Essays on an Old Question*. Leonard Michael Koff and Brenda Deen Schildgen, eds. London: Associated University Presses, 2000, esp. p. 134.

26. Hutcheon, Linda, *A Theory of Parody: The Teachings of Twentieth Century Art Forms*, New York: Methuen, 1985, 6. For scholarship related to *Women's Decameron*, see Ruthchild, Rochelle, "From Russia with Sex," *The Women's Review of Books*, vol. IV, no. 5 (February 1987); Goscilo, Helena, "Women's Wards and Wardens: The Hospital in Contemporary Russian Women's Fiction," *Canadian Woman Studies* 10.4 (1989): 83–86; Kolodziej, Jerzy, "Julia Voznesenskaia's Women with Love and Squalor," *Fruits of Her Plume: Essays on Contemporary Russian Woman's Culture*, Helena Goscilo, ed. Armonk, N.Y.: M.E. Sharpe, 1995; Murav, Harriet, "Engendering the Russian Body Politic," *Genders 22: Postcommunism and the Body Politic*. Ellen E. Barry, ed. New York: NYU Press, 1995; Donovan, Josephine, "Women and the Framed-Novelle: A Tradition of their Own," 22.4 (Summer 1997): 947–980; Furman, Yelena, "'We All Love with the Same Part of the Body, Don't We?': Iuliia Voznesenskaia's *Zhenskii Dekameron*, New Women's Prose, and French Feminist Theory," *Intertexts* 13.1 (2010): 95–114.

27. Whether the doctors on Voznesenskaya's ward are female or male is unclear and irrelevant.

28. Gray, Francine du Plessix, *Soviet Women Walking the Tightrope*, New York: Doubleday, 1989, 131.

29. American novelist Fay Weldon reviewed *Women's Decameron* with the title "The Female Experience—Uncensored." Surely Voznesenskaya influenced Weldon's own *Spa Decameron*, from 2007, which was roundly panned by reviewers who claimed among other things that "mostly the pleasure of the novel comes from its topicality [Skype, no less] and [its] bitchiness." See Body, Kasia, "Sex Makes Your Muscles Softer," *The Telegraph*, October 13, 2007.

30. Murav, "Engendering the Russian Body Politic," 49.

31. As I've argued elsewhere, in *Master and Margarita* (completed 1940) Mikhail Bulgakov represents the psychiatric ward as a place of rest and respite—exactly how Ruthchild sees the medical situation for new mothers in Voznesenskaya. See Brintlinger, Angela, "The Hero in the Madhouse: The Post-Soviet Novel Confronts the Soviet Past," *Slavic Review* 63.1 (Spring 2004): 43–65.

32. Voznesenskaya, Julia, *The Women's Decameron*. W. B. Linton, trans. New York: Henry Holt and Company, 1987, 1. In the Russian version, there are additional comments about how sometimes in a critical introduction the reader learns not only the content of the book, but also the ways in which the author did not understand his own material "because he is influenced by a bourgeois worldview." This is what I have in mind by "arch, dissident" voice. Voznesenskaia, Iulia, *Zhenskii dekameron*, Moscow: Vernisazh, 1992, 3.

33. Weldon, Fay, "The Female Experience—Uncensored," *New York Times Book Review*, October 26, 1986, 9.

34. Steinberg, Sybil, *Publishers Weekly*, August 22, 1986, 78. The conflation of these Soviet sites of abode deserves a treatment all its own.

35. Quoted from Brodsky, Joseph, "The Writer in Prison," *New York Times on the Web,* October 13, 1996, http://movies2.nytimes.com/books/00/09/17/specials/brodsky-prison.html. Last accessed January 25, 2020.

36. Voznesenskaya, *Zhenskii dekameron*, 328; *The Women's Decameron*, 300.

37. Voznesenskaya, *Zhenskii dekameron*, 329; *The Women's Decameron*, 302.

38. Yaffa, Joshua, "A Learned Neighbor," *The New Yorker*, May 13, 2019, 18–24.

39. Blaisdell, Bob, "The Good Doctor: On Maxim Osipov's 'Rock, Paper, Scissors,'" *Los Angeles Review of Books*, April 9, 2019.

40. Quoted from Svetlana Alexievich's preface to Osipov, Maxim, *Rock, Paper, Scissors and Other Stories*. Trans. Alex Fleming, Boris Dralyuk, ed. Preface by Svetlana Alexievich. New York: New York Review of Books, 2019, vii.

41. Osipov, "After Eternity," *Rock, Paper, Scissors and Other Stories*, 235.

WORKS CITED

Blaisdell, Bob. "The Good Doctor: On Maxim Osipov's 'Rock, Paper, Scissors.'" *Los Angeles Review of Books*. April 9, 2019.

Body, Kasia. "Sex Makes Your Muscles Softer." *The Telegraph*. October 13, 2007.

Brintlinger, Angela. "The Hero in the Madhouse: The Post-Soviet Novel Confronts the Soviet Past." *Slavic Review* 63.1 (Spring 2004): 43–65.

Brintlinger, Angela and Ilya Vinitsky, eds. *Madness and the Mad in Russian Culture*. Toronto: University of Toronto Press, 2007.

Brodsky, Joseph. "The Writer in Prison." *New York Times on the Web*. October 13, 1996. http://movies2.nytimes.com/books/00/09/17/specials/brodsky-prison.html. Last accessed January 25, 2020.

Chekhov, Anton. *Anton Chekhov's Selected Stories*, ed. Cathy Popkin. New York: W.W. Norton & Company, 2014.

Chekhov, Anton. *Polnoe sobranie pisem v 12 tomakh*. Moscow: Nauka, 1974–83.

Chekhov, Anton. *Polnoe sobranie sochinenii v 18 tomakh*. Moscow: Nauka, 1974–83.

Donovan, Josephine. "Women and the Framed-Novelle: A Tradition of their Own." *Signs* vol. 22, no. 4 (Summer 1997): 947–980.

Finke, Michael. *Seeing Chekhov: Life and Art*. Cornell UP, 2005.

Furman, Yelena. "'We All Love with the Same Part of the Body, Don't We?': Iuliia Voznesenskaia's *Zhenskii Dekameron*, New Women's Prose, and French Feminist Theory." *Intertexts* 13.1 (2010): 95–114.

Ganim, John M. "Chaucer, Boccaccio, Confession and Subjectivity." In *The Decameron and the Canterbury Tales: New Essays on an Old Question*. Leonard Michael Koff and Brenda Deen Schildgen, eds. London: Associated University Presses, 2000.

Goering, Laura. "'Russian Nervousness': Neurasthenia and National Identity in Nineteenth Century Russia." *Medical History* 47.1 (2003): 23–46.

Goscilo, Helena. "Women's Wards and Wardens: The Hospital in Contemporary Russian Women's Fiction." *Canadian Woman Studies* 10.4 (1989): 83–86.

Gray, Francine du Plessix. *Soviet Women Walking the Tightrope.* New York: Doubleday, 1989.

Hutcheon, Linda. *A Theory of Parody: The Teachings of Twentieth Century Art Forms.* New York: Methuen, 1985.

Jones, Polly. "Diagnosing the Stalinist Sickness: Images of Illness in Aleksandr Bek and Aleksandr Solzhenitsyn." *Modern Language Review* 111.4 (October 2016): 1085–1112.

Kolodziej, Jerzy. "Julia Voznesenskaia's Women with Love and Squalor." *Fruits of Her Plume: Essays on Contemporary Russian Woman's Culture.* Helena Goscilo, ed. Armonk, N.Y.: M.E. Sharpe, 1995. 225–238.

Morrissey, Susan K. "The Economy of Nerves: Health, Commercial Culture and the Self in Late Imperial Russia." *Slavic Review* 69.3 (Fall 2010): 645–675.

Moteiunaite, Ilona. *Vospriiatie iurodstva russkoi literaturoi XIX–XX vekov.* Pskov, 2011.

Murav, Harriet. "Engendering the Russian Body Politic." *Genders 22: Postcommunism and the Body Politic.* Ellen E. Barry, ed. New York: NYU Press, 1995. 32–56.

Osipov, Maxim. *Rock, Paper, Scissors and Other Stories.* Trans. Alex Fleming, Boris Dralyuk, ed. Preface by Svetlana Alexievich. New York: New York Review of Books, 2019.

Pervushin, Nikolai V. "Preliminary Remarks on the Literary Craft of Solzhenitsyn." *Canadian Slavonic Papers*, 13.2 & 3 (1971): 141–146.

Popkin, Cathy. "Doctor without Patients/Man without a Spleen: A Meditation on Chekhov's Practice." *Chekhov the Immigrant: Translating a Cultural Icon.* Ed. Michael C. Finke and Julie de Sherbinin. Bloomington, IN: Slavica, 2007. 219–237.

Reich, Rebecca. *State of Madness: Psychiatry, Literature, and Dissent After Stalin.* Northern Illinois University Press, 2018.

Rothberg, Abram. *Aleksandr Solzhenitsyn: The Major Novels.* Ithaca: Cornell UP, 1971.

Ruthchild, Rochelle. "From Russia with Sex." *The Women's Review of Books*, vol. IV, no. 5 (February 1987).

Sirotkina, Irina. *Diagnosing Literary Genius: A Cultural History of Psychiatry in Russia, 1880–1930.* Baltimore: Johns Hopkins University Press, 2002.

Solzhenitsyn, Alexander. *Cancer Ward.* Nicholas Bethell and David Burg, trans. New York: The Modern Library, 1995.

Solzhenitsyn, Aleksandr. *Rakovyi korpus.* Paris: YMCA Press, 1970.

Smernoff, Susan S. "The Irony of the Doctor as Patient in Chekhov's 'Ward No. 6' and in Solzhenitsyn's 'Cancer Ward.'" *Chekhov's Art of Writing: A Collection of Critical Essays.* Paul Debreczeny and Thomas Eekman, eds. Columbus, OH: Slavica, 1977. 167–179.

Steinberg, Sybil. *Publishers Weekly.* August 22, 1986.

Vidaver, Doris and Maynard M. Cohen. "Vocation: Dr. A. P. Chekhov." *The American Scholar* 55.2 (Spring 1986): 227–233.

Voznesenskaya, Julia. *The Women's Decameron.* W. B. Linton, trans. New York: Henry Holt and Company, 1987.

Voznesenskaia, Iulia. *Zhenskii dekameron.* Moscow: Vernisazh, 1992.

Weales, Gerald. "Chekhov: The Doctor Is In." *The Sewanee Review* 113, no. 2 (2005): 327–332.
Weldon, Fay. "The Female Experience—Uncensored." *New York Times Book Review*, October 26, 1986: 9.
Yaffa, Joshua. "A Learned Neighbor." *The New Yorker*. May 13, 2019: 18–24.

Chapter Nine

Still Alice, Always Elena

Dementia as a World of Possibility

Jehanne Gheith

Miss Agnes was curled up on the sofa in a position that looked anatomically impossible. She had end stage Alzheimer's and, in 2014, I was her hospice social worker.

Over time, I watched Miss Agnes and her husband, James (not their real names), in their daily life: the meals that, increasingly, James had to feed her; the toileting that changed from largely independent to Depends; and the one golden day that the family brought in a hair stylist to cut Miss Agnes's hair. It was a beautiful fall day and they worked on the porch, the daughter calming her mother, the stylist chatting and expertly cutting. That day Miss Agnes stretched out, literally and figuratively. She fully relaxed. I watched Miss Agnes light up for her husband even when she could no longer speak. He told stories about her as a young woman, reminding her of who she had been. And he told stories about before he knew her, when she was a girl, emphasizing that she had been in foster homes and regularly abandoned. He was the keeper of a past she could no longer communicate, but one that still resonated for her; she smiled at the jokes and looked sad at the difficult parts—even when she was largely uncommunicative. James said he would stay with her to the end, and he did that, even when that became complicated.

In time, James needed a few days off in order to sustain the marathon of long-term caregiving that Alzheimer's demands. Medicare provides for respite care for the caregivers of hospice patients and Miss Agnes was transferred from her home to a skilled nursing facility so that James could go on a trip. When their daughter visited the nursing home, she found her mother soaked in urine. I visited Miss Agnes at the nursing home daily. And when she went home, Miss Agnes would often lie with her head in my lap during my visits, a sign of incredible trust.

Most hospices regularly place clinicians where the administration thinks they are most needed. And so, the primary nurse and I were transferred to another area and Miss Agnes's family left hospice shortly after that: they, as many families do, felt attached to particular clinicians and had a hard time making the transition to new clinical staff. My experience with Miss Agnes and her family—and many others I had as a hospice social worker—taught me about dementia/Alzheimer's[1] and how we handle them as a culture. I learned that the woman I saw in Miss Agnes was not who her husband and daughter saw; that relationship is possible in and through dementia (this should be obvious, but in our society it is not); that families can work with grace and strength to care for those with Alzheimer's or dementia; and that the medical system, including hospice, fails people with dementia—and their families—all the time.

I am both a social worker and a professor of Russian literature and I have done a lot of work with hospice. The social work side of my professional life focuses now on private practice, primarily with those who are ill or grieving. The two vocations work seamlessly together (well, most of the time). The way I understand the patients and families I work with is shaped by my immersion in Russian literature and, in turn, my understanding of Russian literature is now informed by my clinical work. Both Russian literature and my work as a therapist give me ways to hold difficult stories and to use the transformative power of those stories to make sense of dynamics that people find puzzling or painful. I have learned that stories affect us on many levels—and that is the central point of this essay. Here I explore how the stories we tell about dementia affect how we understand and treat people with memory loss. Can close analysis of literature, stories, affect how we understand and interact with people who live with dementia—both patients and caregivers? I believe that it can, that looking deeply into the stories we tell has the potential to transform our understanding and behavior. I see it every day in my clinical practice and in my teaching.

In recounting the case study of Miss Agnes (one form of storytelling), I show the individual pain of dementia and the poor healthcare available for it, even in the Duke system which is widely considered to provide high quality care. My teaching also focuses on dementia as a huge, predictable, social problem that we, as a society, are not addressing well. In 2019, over 5.5 million people in the US have Alzheimer's and there are many other forms of dementia. It is predicted that by 2050 over 13 million people in the US will have Alzheimer's.[2] We should be preparing for this great wave; we are not. As Ashton Applewhite, Atul Gawande, and others have shown,[3] in this society, we refuse to look at the issue of aging and of memory loss, as if that refusal to see will make it go away.

So what can novels have to do with the world of dementia on the individual and social level?

Performer, author, and teacher Kali Quinn, in conversation with my students, made it clear that we are not willing to look at this problem partly because of what Quinn calls The Empathy Wall. In this essay, I will argue that novels can help us scale that Wall,[4] and that novels provide a way to understand dementia in more complex ways than much of the clinical literature allows. Novels (and the other arts) allow us to imagine the inner world of dementia and its impact on families, in a way that clinical literature struggles to do. They do this by inviting, perhaps even requiring, readers to inhabit these worlds over time. Stories, as Rebecca Solnit, Janelle Taylor, Dana Walroth, and others have shown, can shape how we live with dementia—as patients, caregivers, and as a society.[5] These authors suggest the limits of our current stories, as does Mary Hume, who argues that our cultural stories about dementia show how our societal value of economic productivity leads us to devalue those who can no longer be "productive."[6] We need bigger, more complex stories about dementia.

While clinicians and scholars including Mary Hume, Judith Jordan, Tom Kitwood, Stephen Post, and others have shown how working with narrative can help dementia patients and their caregivers, I, like Taylor, Solnit, and others, want to suggest that the stories we tell about dementia go beyond aid to patients and caregivers. They also affect how we more broadly see the disease, creating cultural stories with real social effects. Taylor argues that, in the US, the default genre for Alzheimer stories is horror. In this essay, I will explore two very different novels about significant memory loss, mining them as new stories, stories that move beyond the "horror" of Alzheimer's that Taylor describes.

Both Liudmila Ulitskaia's *The Kukotsky Case* (*Kazus Kukotskogo,* published in 2000, translated by Diane Nemec Ignashev, as *The Kukotsky Enigma*, in 2016) and *Still Alice* by Lisa Genova (published in 2007) have won wide recognition.[7] These two novels are immensely, wonderfully complicated and they do very different work. *Still Alice* places Alice, a Harvard professor, at the center of the story which takes place from 2003 to 2005. In *The Kukotsky Case*, Elena is part of a family saga—not her family of origin, but one she joins by marriage: the Kukotskys, who have been a family of doctors since the seventeenth century. The time period covered in *The Kukotsky Case* is the early twentieth century to the 1990s—just pre-Soviet to just post-Soviet—with the main action taking place in the middle of the Soviet period. Elena's story is one small part of a much larger tale of family and country. It is significant, though, that although the two novels depict memory loss very differently, they both end with generational continuation: Alice with her daughters and grandson; Elena (and others) becoming aware of her great grandson's birth.

STORIES ABOUT DEMENTIA

Janelle Taylor's essay "Recognition, Caring, and Dementia" frames the issues around story and dementia beautifully. She argues that two of the most powerful and widespread stories we tell about dementia in the US are the gothic story and the zombie story. The gothic: "A person you love, and to whom you are bound by unbreakable ties, turns out to be someone you do not know at all, who does not 'care' about you and may even seek to harm you: this is the classic gothic plot."[8] And the zombie story: the person you love is gone but their body lives on. As she explores her mother's "progressive dementia," Taylor seeks to move beyond these two stories and show how the person with dementia is now living a different, but potentially rich, life. And further, that the telling and retelling of gothic and zombie stories in various keys leads to and maintains problematic medical, personal, and social consequences for people with dementia, their caregivers, and society more broadly. We need better stories.

Taylor contends both that our cultural stories do important work and that we can change them. Her article demonstrates that people with dementia can express recognition and care in non-verbal ways and differently—but no less powerfully—from how the person expressed them before they developed dementia. By taking us through how often people ask the question, "Does she still recognize you?" and asking what cultural work that question does, Taylor demonstrates that the way we look at Alzheimer's and dementia needs both better stories and new interpretive strategies. Her mother expressed a desire to "keep all the cares together." Taylor explores that as metaphor, arguing that as a goal, keeping the things and people you care about together works far better than considering dementia as only loss. She argues that we are afraid that those with dementia no longer care about us but that, in fact, they do, they just show it differently than they did before the memory loss. Taylor asks us to consider: How do people continue to recognize and care when their cognitive function declines radically? Why do we tend to see this disease as only loss? What do the gothic/zombie/loss stories allow and what do they prevent? What are we afraid of? Perhaps, she suggests, the problem lies in the eye of the caregiver or the eye of those of us who, for now, do not have Alzheimer's or dementia.[9] And perhaps it lies, at least in part, in the stories we tell.[10]

Both *The Kukotsky Case* and *Still Alice* provide extended reflections on these questions in novel form. And both seek to change common cultural stories, and to "keep the cares together" though they do this in very different ways. The epigraphs to each novel are revealing. *The Kukotsky Case* begins with a quotation from Simone Weil: "Truth is on the side of death." And death comes into the novel in many ways: in fact, *The Kukotsky Case* can be read as being about the liminal space between life and death where death—and disease—are not the enemy. The epigraph to *Still Alice* reads:

> Even then, more than a year earlier, there were neurons in her head, not far from her ears, that were being strangled to death, too quietly for her to hear them. Some would argue that things were going so insidiously wrong that the neurons themselves initiated events that would lead to their own destruction. Whether it was molecular murder or cellular suicide, they were unable to warn her of what was happening before they died.

From the beginning, then, Genova positions Alzheimer's as primarily a disease and in quite violent terms: "strangle," "murder," "suicide"—terms that show a clear resonance with Taylor's horror story of Alzheimer's. Alice is a renowned scholar at Harvard and throughout much of the novel, we see Alzheimer's primarily as loss. Brilliant thinking has been a major part of Alice's personal and professional life, a part of her life that is threatened by her early onset Alzheimer's. Initially, Alice hopes she has a brain tumor because that would be better than Alzheimer's, thus showing the profound fear that many of us have around issues of memory loss. Alice gradually loses memories and objects, like her Blackberry (which her husband, John, finds in the freezer) and eventually her career, as she is no longer able to lecture, research, work with graduate students. As Alice's disease progresses, there is also a growing, painful distance between Alice and John. She undergoes memory tests, takes medications, and receives medical care. And yet, Genova tells a positive story, too: At the end of the novel, Alice cannot remember her daughter Lydia's name but she relates more lovingly to her daughter than before she had Alzheimer's. And, although Alice can no longer work, she delights in her grandson and is able to relate to emotions even though (or partly because?) she has lost much of what used to define her identity. In the novel, Genova depicts Alice as a full person—in some ways a fuller person than before—even through the loss of her memory. This is a story we do not often tell: that a person with dementia continues internal growth. In a complicated move, Genova both positions readers in the horror story of Alzheimer's and moves us beyond it.

In *The Kukotsky Case,* Ulitskaia does not ever consider Alzheimer's as "horror story"; instead, she offers radically new possibilities for understanding the internal world of dementia. First, Ulitskaia embeds the story of memory loss in a larger field of family and country, where Elena is not the only central character; her trajectory is one thread in multiple stories. And Elena's "dementia" is not discussed as a disease. The person she plans to talk with about her memory loss is a priest, not a doctor; she faces no medical tests, no medicines. While this is partly a result of the different time periods and cultures that the two novels inhabit, it is more than that. In *The Kukotsky Case*, we can't be certain that Elena's memory loss is dementia: but her writing of notes to herself early in the novel, her gradual descent into loss of memory, and her growing need for others to care for her lead me to be comfortable in saying that we, in the West, would call this dementia. And the fact that Ulitskaia does not move to pathologize memory loss is significant, as it presents different possibilities for what dementia can be. As I will consider in this essay, the two novels together explore the territory of Taylor's article, the zombie and gothic stories; both novels create better stories and more interpretive possibilities, and new stories for how to understand and live with diseases (or changes?) of memory.

STILL ALICE

Alice's story is complex—it is multiple stories, really, as all powerful stories of family and disease are. The main action is centered on one individual, Alice, and readers are often inside her consciousness. Over the course of the novel, she moves from being a highly successful Harvard professor to not knowing what the word "commencement" means; this process is sometimes heartbreaking for both characters and readers. We see Alice lose words, not remembering, for example, the words for "cream cheese," naming it "white butter"[11] instead (an act that could be seen as loss or as creative—or both). Loss is described in another key as Genova explores the effect of the disease on caregivers: Alice's husband John is not able to be present with Alice as her Alzheimer's progresses, but their daughters are able to grow with Alice into the disease.

The complex intertwining of stories of loss and gain continues throughout the novel. Even fairly late in the novel, Alice is active; she starts a support group for those with early onset Alzheimer's and she delivers a moving keynote speech to the annual Dementia Care Conference of the Alzheimer's Association. And as the title indicates, even at the end of the novel, when she cannot remember her daughter's name, she is STILL Alice, creative and generous, a person capable of giving love and worthy of receiving it. Each of these stories of growth also incorporate loss: this is the tension of

Alzheimer's. Genova tells the stories of the losses and gains of Alzheimer's, both staying within and moving beyond Taylor's zombie and gothic stories; she helps readers to empathize with Alice and her caregivers, showing how Alice "keep(s) the cares together" and helping readers to do that, to begin to care differently about those who have Alzheimer's.

Genova builds much empathy for Alice into the novel. But there is, for me at least, an undertaste, seen even in the title: *Still Alice*. In one way, the title is beautiful: even with all the cognitive decline, at the end of the novel, she is Alice, a creative person, deserving of love and capable of care. And yet, in another way, this "still" is part of the problem. Here is how Taylor describes the "stills" indicating that there is a drop of poison in them: the "stills" assume that "our" criteria are the right ones:

> One can measure the advance of dementia by the "stills." The social worker will ask the *still* questions: Does she *still* feed herself? *Good!* Still chew? *Good!* Still toilet? Well, that's to be expected. And we have ours: Still like to dress up? Get her hair done? Her nails? Still hang on to her French and German? Yes, a few words, pretty good accent. Still play the piano? Oh yes, the "Anniversary Waltz," over and over. Still like parties? Oh-ho, *does she ever!*[12]

Taylor also notes that the "stills" are matched by the "firsts"—the first time that a person with Alzheimer's repeats the same question in a short space of time, the first time they try to do some daily act and cannot. Yet, she adds:

> it bears saying that not all of the "stills" and the "firsts" necessarily tell a grim story of unremitting decline, loss, humiliation, and disappearance. Despite all the changes she has been through my mother "still" is in many ways the cheerful, affectionate person I have always known her to be. . . . And for my part . . . some of the "firsts" have been tender moments that I cherish. The "first" time since my early childhood that my Mom and I walked down the street holding hands . . .[13]

Genova's title, then, expresses the tightrope of Alzheimer's. It indicates both that Alice remains defined by usual societal standards of what is STILL important but it also reclaims something vital: that though Alice acts differently due to Alzheimer's, she remains herself in crucial ways.

Medicalization of Alzheimer's

Treating Alzheimer's as a medical disease is so normative in the US that we forget that the medicalization of memory loss is not the only possible approach. In her novel, Genova explores what conceptualizing Alzheimer's primarily in medical terms means for patients and families. She begins with the medical—as we have seen in the epigraph and its image of murderous or suicidal neurons in Alice's brain. Alice goes to a doctor early on and, although her husband John votes against it, she decides to go with her doctor's recommendation and undergoes a clinical trial of the (fictional) drug Amylix, which, we learn at the end of the novel, has no significant effect on the disease. Would she have fared better if she had decided on the treatment that John wanted her to do? It is unknowable, but John weeps as he reads about the failure of the trial. He ultimately put his faith in the medical establishment because he understands the world, as many people in the US do, through medical and scientific stories.

The way Genova tells Alice's story depicts medicalization of Alzheimer's as having its uses but also as having significant downsides: scientific discourse, in Genova's depiction, is not enough and cannot bear all the weight we put on it. We see this in Alice's visits to the doctor over time, which show her increasing inability to draw a clock accurately and to remember the facts that the doctor thinks she should remember (e.g., "can you spell the word *water* backwards,"[14] "name as many vegetables/four-legged animals as you can").[15] The doctor sees Alice as being resourceful and creative, but John sees only her diminishment.[16] Alice herself finds the visits painful both because of John's response and because she feels "ruthlessly pummeled by so many tests."[17] In these clinical visits, we see John begin to speak for Alice, talking about her as if she cannot understand. Sometimes she cannot, or it takes her more time to get the point and Alice feels hurt by his frustration with her. She also experiences emotional pain when she cannot accomplish the tests easily. Through this portrayal, Genova suggests that the medicalization of Alzheimer's often affects both those with the disease and their caregivers in negative ways: the measurement of memory loss doesn't seem to help anyone involved. On the other hand, the medical context does give Alice a chance to start a support group and the opportunity to use her talents and help others in her keynote speech to the Alzheimer's Association. Alice's doctor also recommends that John seek support for his role as caregiver—but John does not follow up on this suggestion. Medicalization of dementia, then, is depicted as normative, and sometimes useful, but also problematic. In the US, the novel shows, dementia tests are the measure of cognitive ability and, for most people, there is no room for acceptance of another reality. That is very different, as we will see, in Ulitskaia's novel, where the possibilities, rather than the losses, of dementia are highlighted.

Caregiving

Through the character of John, we experience Alzheimer's through the eyes of the caregiver. John tries to support Alice but cannot bear to see her diminished. He goes to all of her medical appointments, researches cures, and advocates for her in the medical system. He tries to run with Alice even though he hates running. He gets videos of her favorite books when she can no longer read them (heartbreaking for someone who has lived a life reading and writing books). But what Alice most wants is John's presence and this he cannot give her. Instead, he spends more and more time at work. Most poignantly: They have sabbatical years approaching and Alice wants desperately for them to spend this year, potentially the last year of her life, together. But John chooses instead to accept a job in New York rather than stay in Cambridge with Alice:

> I don't think I can do it, Alice. I'm sorry, I just don't think I can take being home for a whole year, just sitting and watching what this disease is stealing from you. I can't take watching you not knowing how to get dressed and not knowing how to work the television. If I'm in lab, I don't have to watch you sticking Post-it notes on all the cabinets and doors. I can't just stay home and watch you get worse. It kills me.[18]

Alice rightly comments that the disease is actually killing her, and not him. But the point here is that John sees Alice's disease as only stealing from her and he can't bear it. And so he cannot give her the gift of presence.

Genova highlights John's inability to be present by showing how Alice and her daughter Lydia become closer through Alice's memory loss. At the very end of the novel, Lydia asks her mother to listen to a monologue for a play that Lydia is rehearsing. She asks Alice to say what she feels as she listens. Alice says:

> "I feel love. It's about love." The actress [Alice's name for Lydia now] squealed, rushed over to Alice and smiled, every crease of her face delighted.
> "Did I get it right?" asked Alice.
> "You did, Mom. You got it exactly right."[19]

This is the end of the novel and is especially moving because Lydia and Alice struggled to relate to one another when Alice had her full cognitive function. Genova suggests here that it is through the experience of memory loss that Alice learns to inhabit emotion and, so, discovers a new way of "keeping the cares together."

John's story suggests that we need different kinds of supports for caregivers of dementia and Alzheimer's, because caregiving is isolating and, perhaps, also because our cultural stories around the disease are so limited and limiting. In Taylor's terms, John sees only the zombie and gothic stories—the diminishment. As anyone who has done caregiving for people with dementia knows, it can be deeply wrenching to watch someone change, lose the capacity to communicate as they used to, and to be unable to care for their own basic needs. But, I wonder: would we, would John move so easily to "horror" and diminishment if other stories about the disease were more easily available? I can't help but believe that because our stories about Alzheimer's are so one-dimensional, they limit our capacity to see more than the pain. The pain is heartbreakingly real. But what if we could also see the creativity within? What if that were a story we told more directly, more loudly? That is: if our culture told other stories about dementia, more complex and nuanced stories, telling of inner worlds and difference, even stories of recreation and recovery, and not just a tale of loss,[20] could John have gained a vocabulary for staying with Alice? And perhaps, if there were stories about presence rather than medicalization, for example, John could have accepted the support he would need to stay with Alice rather than move to New York? That is, would people who respond like John be better able to remain present with Alzheimer's if they had access to the stories Genova, Ulitskaia, or Taylor tell?

By indicating the limits of our current stories about Alzheimer's, as well as by depicting Alice as continuing to be loving and generative throughout the novel and the disease progression, Genova makes room for the possibility that dementia may also hold potential, may hold possibilities as well as perils. And that is the story that Ulitskaia tells in an even bigger key.

THE KUKOTSKY CASE OR "WHERE IS MY LIFE TAKING ME AND WHAT IS IT TRYING TO TELL ME?"

While the plot of *The Kukotsky Case* is not really the point of the novel, I will give a brief plot orientation to provide context for understanding Elena's journey through memory loss. Pavel Alekseevich Kukotsky and Elena Georgievna meet during wartime evacuation in Siberia when Elena comes down with extreme peritonitis. As Elena hovers between life and death Kukotsky, a doctor, performs the life-saving operation. At the time, Elena is married, with a daughter Tanya, but she and Kukotsky come together as a couple.[21] He becomes a loving father to Tanya and eventually, Pavel and Elena marry. Kukotsky is a doctor who advocates for legalizing abortion and this causes a major rift between the couple as Elena believes abortion is a sin; this rift is central in the family story. Her love of Tanya is elemental and clear, and is a motivating force for Elena throughout the novel. The family also includes Vasilisa, a domestic helper who has a long history with Elena, and Toma, a schoolmate of Tanya's, whom the Kukotskys take into their home after Toma's mother dies of a botched abortion.

Fairly early in the novel, but after the couple has become estranged, Elena begins writing notebooks because she is having difficulty with her memory and wants to remember important parts of her life for herself and so that she can pass them on to her daughter Tanya. Elena writes:

> My life in and of itself is so insignificant and I myself am so insignificant that it never would have occurred to me to write anything down, were it not for the fact that my memory is getting worse and worse. It needs some sort of external reinforcement: smells, sounds, objects, that elicit memories, pointers, references. . . . [ellipses in original] So let there be at least this little notebook, and when my memory fails entirely, I will be able to look at it and remember.

She wants to "excavate" her life "like an archeologist" and asks: "where is it [my life] taking me and what is it trying to tell me?' And she adds:

> The most horrifying thing is that my brain has become like an old porcelain cup: it's filled with tiny cracks. My thoughts suddenly cut off, lose themselves, and it take a long time to pick up their trail. Periods when I drop out.[22] Sometimes the image of a person takes on a life separate from the name of its owner. A person you know well . . . suddenly you can't remember their name. . . . Or . . . you remember a name, but not the person behind it.[23]

Elena continues: "Deep in my heart I suspect that this is the beginning of some terrible disease. I just wrote that and now am entirely convinced of it."[24] And she notes that her mother's older sister "reverted to childhood" [25] when she got old: "It's awful: your whole life then becomes senseless. If a person has forgotten her own life—her parents, and children, and loves, joys, and losses—then what was the point of living?"[26] Elena then adds something of great significance: she thinks all people "drop out" in this way, but it is so difficult to describe that we don't talk about these moments where time does not exist, what she calls "border crossings."[27] This is the one place in the novel where Elena names memory loss as disease, and even here, her commentary normalizes the phenomenon: we are all a little bit demented. Or at least, in Elena's formulation, we all can relate to what it means to lose your memory as we all already have moments where we "drop out" of everyday reality and linear time.

Elena relates the experience of "border crossings" to death. She notes: "I'm talking about the border between everyday life and various other conditions I'm acquainted with, but that are as difficult to describe as death. What can a person who has never died say about dying? But it seems to me that each time you drop out of everyday life you die a little bit."[28] She is afraid, she says, not because of the fear of not existing, but because she cannot see the laws that govern the transition. She follows this statement with a story that illustrates her point: memories of her grandmother and grandfather and a time when as a girl, Elena became ill and went into a "spinning blackness" and ended up with a sense of "eternity," in a space without light or shadow, that is called both "the shadow of death" and "the middle world."[29] While this realm is unwelcoming, and frightening, it also brings gifts. It is a world that is separate from, but related to the everyday—and it is not something that Elena wants to avoid. "Dropping out" may be painful, but Elena began to experience it when she was a child and she accepts it as a rich part of life as it continues into her adulthood.

There are, then, many indicators that Elena has the classical signs of what we[30] would call dementia: she loses names, she can't follow threads of conversations, and her family has a history of memory loss; she later gets disoriented and cannot find her way home; again, a common symptom of "dementia." At the end of the novel, her memory loss is even more clear: she is "dropped out" most of the time and has rarer moments of what we would usually call lucidity. But, in her first notebook, written when she was about forty, Elena approaches the experience of memory loss primarily in the context of trying to understand her life: "Where is it taking me and what is it trying to tell me?"[31] She is mostly curious about memory lapses rather than frightened by them.

Memory Loss and the Third Dimension

By profession, Elena is a drafter and she likes to be able to see objects multi-dimensionally, top, bottom, and center. Three views. She also experiences waking life, dream life, and something in between that she calls the third dimension/realm/condition[32] which she sometimes names the "middle world," a place we may all "drop out" into. In this dimension, she sees her grandmother, who has died—but it is not, Elena argues, a dream. While the elements of dream world and third dimension often overlap, this third state is the world Elena "drops out" into[33] when she exhibits what we would call dementia. And this middle world is a state of being where past, present, and future are one.

Elena describes this third dimension in relation to her profession, noting: "Waking reality and dreams: they're like the front and back sides of the same cloth. And what about that third state? Is it like a top view in mechanical drawing?"[34] What Elena calls "external reality" pales in importance beside the realities of dream world and the third dimension. She notes: "Over time, with increasing experience, I have learned how to distinguish one [state] from the other almost infallibly. In the usual daytime world things are totally deprived of mystery and their real content."[35] She considers the world of dreams, too, as deep and rich sources of life: "What I see—what's told to me and shown to me in my dreams—is much richer and more significant that what I can put to paper. I have a wonderful spatial imagination, professional. Probably I am particularly sensitive to space, and for that reason have found myself in its mysterious back alleys, like that 'middle world.'"[36] The richest life, it appears, is lived in these "mysterious back alleys," in the middle world and in dreams, which, for Elena, are the source of meaning and mystery, arguably more real than daytime reality.

After preparing readers through Elena's discussion of this third realm, Ulitskaia then offers us direct experience of it in Part II of the novel. The context for this second section of the book is important: Elena visits a priest, intending to talk about her memory loss, but instead ends up discussing her daughter Tanya. After the visit, Elena gets lost on the way home (this happens to Alice in Genova's novel, too). An unidentified acquaintance sees Elena home where she falls asleep in her chair. Part I ends and we move into the dreamworld? Third state? Increasing dementia? of Part II. This section can be read in any of these ways—and most fruitfully, it can be read in all of these ways.

The Third Realm: A Better World?

Part II begins: "The sand, picked up by a stream of air, rang lightly as it struck against the transparent stalks of the dry, brittle plants. . . ."[37] And we know we are not in Moscow anymore. This sand world has a "multidimensional" set of coordinates,[38] each individual has their own coordinates of time and space and some locations are not visible to others. The multiple variations of time include: "hot time, cold time, historical, metahistorical, personal, abstract, accentuated, reverse, and many, many other [kinds of time]."[39] Temperature and light, too, are ambiguous: "It was neither cold nor hot. It grew neither darker nor lighter; it was early dusk and it seemed as if nothing here intended to change."[40] In this world, many of the ways we usually orient—like time, temperature, and contact with others—are not available to the characters. This is a profoundly disorienting world—both for characters and for readers.

The characters in this realm are named The Judean, Skinhead, the Professor, Longhair, and Katya.[41] The reader experiences this world through the eyes of the Newling.[42] It gradually becomes clear these characters stand in for people we meet in other parts of the novel: The Newling is a version of Elena; Skinhead, an overlay of her husband Pavel (Kukotsky); The Judean, his friend Goldberg; Longhair is related to Sergei, who only appears later in the novel. Many of the main themes of the novel such as abortion are raised in Part II in a different key and, I would argue, in a way that helps us scale the empathy wall and inhabit—at least a little—the world of someone with profound memory loss.

In this world, Elena experiences a kind of newness. Her body is different; at first encased in some muddy material which falls off, leaving "new young skin" like that of an infant.[43] This is a positive experience: "how wonderful, she thought. I'm like new." And she's not surprised; this feels right and good—this inner realm she inhabits while being "dropped out" of the "waking reality" of the novel. "She ran her hand over her face and hair: everything was her own, yet everything was changed. . . ." A little further down the page: "Walking felt good. Effortless. She was young and light. Everything was absolutely as it should be, although not at all like what she had prepared herself for so long."[44] The Newling then experiences this sandworld as sometimes monotonous, but full of vitality and new possibilities. There are no zombie or gothic stories here; instead, this is a story of new life.

It also turns out that what is unfixable or problematic in Moscow is healed in the third dimension. In the sand world, for example, unborn children appear several times. At one point "the aborted ones . . . ripen and reemerge,"[45] with Skinhead (Kukotsky) as their "midwife."[46] Given that, in the everyday world Elena and Kukotsky fight bitterly over abortion, it is significant that in this middle world, they work together and he gives life to the unborn ones. Several other examples: The Judean says that all in this realm are "saints";[47] one character who cannot read in the outside world can read in the middle world;[48] a third character, Katya (perhaps related to Toma, who lives with the Kukotskys in Moscow), is able to master Landscape Architecture here where she could not in Moscow. The most important healing comes between Skinhead and the Newling who at the end of Part II gradually surface as Pavel[49] and Elena.[50] The two come together emotionally and physically in the third realm in a way that never happens in their Moscow life. Much like the world of dreams, the desert world makes right what the daily world cannot.

In a complicated move, Ulitskaia also suggests that Elena's memory loss functions as predictive dream and even that, in a sense, she has—probably not consciously—chosen memory loss as a way not to know that a tragedy will befall her daughter. That is, Ulitskaia intimates that Elena's intuition is so strong that she knows something terrible will happen to Tanya, and she chooses to retreat into the third dimension in order not to know. This is a strong suggestion, daringly told. To quickly sketch some of the evidence for this: Elena meets Longhair in the sand world with his "Selmer" instrument before her daughter Tanya meets Sergei (the love of her life) in what most would call the "real world" of the novel. The connection is never made explicitly, but as Tanya is about to die, Sergei, who has had long hair, serenades her on his Selmer saxophone.[51] And after Tanya's death, Kukotsky wonders: "might Elena have departed for her empty, enigmatic, mad world so as never to learn about what her prophetic heart had glimpsed long ago . . . ?" (ellipses in text).[52] This is dizzying, but here again, Ulitskaia merges time: before Tanya has even met Sergei, Elena already intuited both Sergei's presence in Tanya's life and her daughter's early death. Time is not linear. Coordinates are multiple. We all "drop out."

Ulitskaia implies that memory loss may be refuge as well as loss, may be possibility as well as peril, may be better, in some instances, than retaining full cognition. That memory loss may be the preferred option is surprising and complicated. We are so afraid of dementia in our culture[53] that we may shrink from Ulitskaia's intimation that losing one's memory may not always be the worst option. I do not say this lightly; nor do I think that Ulitskaia makes the suggestion lightly. It is the great gift of literary/artistic understanding, that Ulitskaia can evoke this possibility—that memory loss may function as protection—without proof or insisting, rather raising it as a question, a possibility, a kind of haunting.[54]

While I wonder if some may think that Ulitskaia is fantasizing or engaging in a kind of blaming the person with dementia for retreating into forgetting, we know that certain kinds of trauma do predispose people to memory loss so that even here, Ulitskaia's rendering fits with the scholarship: memory loss can be what our bodies do to protect us. Ulitskaia is trained as a scientist, specifically she has degrees in genetics and biochemistry and she has conducted medical research. I am not arguing that she is necessarily consciously aware of the scholarship of trauma as she writes, but rather that, just as the fact that Chekhov's medical understanding of the body is clear throughout his fiction (e.g., "In the Ravine," "Sleepy"), Ulitskaia's orientation toward scientific inquiry and curiosity inflects all her work, including how she presents Elena—and the works she asks of readers—in *The Kukotsky Case.*[55]

In Part II, Ulitskaia forces the reader into the middle realm, to wander in confusion for about eighty pages. It is a daring move. She requires readers to experience life in Elena's third dimension, in a world where coordinates are multiple and there is such a thing as hot time. If we are willing to go with her, we "drop out" into this world. Wandering through the sand world, readers don't know how to evaluate what is real or important; our usual categories for understanding don't apply. It is profoundly uncomfortable to not understand, to be unsure of what is real and unreal, and how one evaluates the difference. And yet, by immersing us in this third realm, Ulitskaia ensures that we so thoroughly experience the disorientation of memory loss that we cannot think of Elena as simply diminished or lesser unless we deploy heavy defensive strategies. And, further, in the vision of memory loss that Ulitskaia creates, there is no loss of control and personality in the ways that we think about it in the US. Rather, she presents "dementia" as a journey, as an opening to another world, a world full of possibility rather than of degeneration. It is a realm that involves pain and uncertainty, but it is also a realm of relationship, growth, protection, learning, care, and healing.

Ending in Possibility

Elena's being, and her capacity for deep care and meaning, connects the worlds of dream, third dimension, and daytime reality together. To use Taylor's language, even when we return to Moscow and Elena is deep in memory loss, she, like Alice, "keeps the cares together." At the end of the novel, Elena is living with Toma, whom she raised. But it is Tanya's daughter, Zhenya, Elena's granddaughter, who comes over to bathe and care for her. Elena and Zhenya have a lovely relationship of mutual care. And, even though Elena is "dropped out" most of the time, she remains connected to the world in the ways that Taylor suggests will be true. When Zhenya gives birth, even though Elena has not been told, she has a dream of people past and present, living and dead, her relatives and the Kukotskys on a balcony—more people than could possibly fit into that space. In her dream, they are all alive. And there is "a girl resembling Tanechka or Zhenya or Tomochka, with an infant in her arms . . . this infant . . . belonged to them all, and they to it. And Elena Georgievena sobbed with perfect happiness, just a tiny bit amazed that she could sense both the salty sweetness of her tears and her total disembodiment. . . ."[56] She has this dream just as, in many different parts of the world, relatives and friends are learning of Zhenya's son's birth. In this way, Ulitskaia depicts Elena as remaining in touch with the essence of life, connecting everyone, living and dead: she is, at least internally, "keeping the cares together."

Externally, Elena is living a very diminished life. Those she lives with—Toma and her husband—do not relate well to her. In fact, Toma has recently moved Elena into the servant's pantry. It would be easy to see Elena's life as evidence of Taylor's gothic or zombie story. And yet Elena remains connected to those she loves through her dreams. Again, Ulitskaia gives readers a way to see into the world of dementia as a world of inner possibility rather than simply of loss. She also suggests here that caregivers of those with dementia need to have a capacity for imagination as Toma's poor care of Elena is partly a result of Toma's lack of imagination. Throughout the novel, Toma regularly misinterprets stories; she is too literal to understand nuance or mystery. Toma cannot treat Elena better, Ulitskaia suggests, partly because of her limited fund of stories and imagination. This argument may be difficult to follow, but the important point here is that Ulitskaia shows that lack of imagination results in poor care of those who suffer from memory loss. Elena, even though she is "dropped out," is far better able to "keep the cares together" than Toma, who has no memory loss. We need then, not only better stories about what memory loss means, but better imaginations in order to work well with it.

BACK TO MISS AGNES

So what does knowing the stories of Alice and Elena, both fictional characters, have to do with Miss Agnes with whom I began this essay? Ulitskaia's vision—and to a certain extent Genova's—shaped my understanding of Miss Agnes's world. They helped me to see that Miss Agnes faced a world of possibilities I could not imagine (a sand world, but not a lesser world), I believe that this helped me to be gentle and respectful with her in a way that resonated with her and with her family. When I sat with Miss Agnes, sometimes with her head in my lap, I wasn't thinking that she was inert and cognitively impaired; I was thinking that there was something important happening within her, that she lived in a world that I did not have access to. And this showed, I think: Miss Agnes and the family responded well to me because my understanding of what it means to be human is fundamentally shaped by Russian literature and, in this case, by Ulitskaia's presentation of memory loss. And, because, as noted in the opening case study, Miss Agnes had experienced early abandonment and trauma, I thought about how Ulitskaia depicts Elena's journey as both painful and fruitful and wondered how the pain was shaped for Miss Agnes in her current world of Alzheimer's. My reading of Ulitskaia—and other Russian literature[57]—gave me a capacity to sit with and be present to this family's difficult stories—and to see the patients and families I worked with as immensely complex, part of a more expansive reality.

CONCLUSION

I hope that through my reading of these two novels I have shown how deeply inhabiting literary works can develop new vocabulary, new ways of understanding and interpreting the worlds of memory loss, and that I have begun to make available some fresh stories, stories in which dementia may be not only loss, but also offer possibilities. Reshaping cultural stories is slow work. But I believe it accomplishes the deep work of change in a longer-lasting way than many apparently quicker fixes and that it can affect how we relate to one another and to memory loss in profound and nuanced ways.

I will close by briefly returning to the two novels. *Still Alice* is an important work of fiction that brings us into the world of Alzheimer's in realistic and touching ways, showing Alice's story as one of disintegration and discovery.

It is far more accessible than *The Kukotsky Case*. Ulitskaia's novel demands and rewards multiple readings; it is multi-layered, offering a dizzying array of interpretive choices. And *Kukotsky* shows that the world of dementia exists all around us and that we drop in and out of it all the time. This novel has no Empathy Wall; the veil between the worlds of memory and memory loss, life and death, past, present, and future is gossamer and we move between them continually. *Still Alice* also rewards multiple readings, but much of the novel can be "gotten" in one thorough reading; unlike *The Kukotsky Case* it is not a palimpsest. Its genius is different: Genova offers the reader deep insight and empathy into the world of Alzheimer's without requiring so much work of the reader.

Together, the two novels undo the zombie and gothic stories. They challenge "the horror of Alzheimer's" and invite us to look anew at people with profound memory loss. Both Genova and Ulitskaia suggest new interpretive possibilities by inviting readers to inhabit the inner worlds of the characters of Alice and Elena. This is, in its way, a revolutionary act, locating the problem not in the "disease" but in our interpretation of it, or, at least, in some combination of "disease" and interpretation. And, as the endings of both novels reveal, the authors emphasize what Taylor calls "keeping the cares together," through intergenerational healing. Through her dreams, Ulitskaia's Elena remains connected to her daughter Tanya, and to her wider family. Genova, too, depicts Alice's creativity throughout her memory loss, and she stresses that a new life with those who have dementia is possible if one has the capacity to move outside traditional narratives about Alzheimer's. Those who do so will see an Alice who cannot say her daughter Lydia's name, but who is able to be immensely present in love, as the last lines of the novel ("it's about love," "you got it right, Mom") make clear.

As for Miss Agnes and others like her, I wonder: if the stories about dementia that we told were different, would she have been treated better at the nursing home? Would her caregivers have gotten more support if they had alternative stories, a broader vocabulary, multiple interpretive strategies? Would we even structure our care for people with dementia differently—if we thought, along with Ulitskaia and Genova, that people with dementia have something big to give us, a world of possibility?

NOTES

1. Throughout, I will use the term "dementia" as it can cover both Alzheimer's and dementia.

2. See the information available at https://www.alz.org/media/Documents/facts-and-figures-2018-r.pdf.

3. Applewhite, Ashton, *This Chair Rocks: A Manifesto against Ageism,* Self-published by Networked Books, 2016; Power, G. Allen, *Dementia beyond Drugs: Changing the Culture of Care.* 2d ed. Baltimore, MD: Health Professions Press, Inc, 2017; Taylor, Janelle S., "On Recognition, Caring, and Dementia," *Medical Anthropology Quarterly* 22.4 (2008): 313–335.

4. This is true of the arts, humanities, and performance more generally, but here I will discuss only novels.

5. Solnit, Rebecca, *The Faraway Nearby,* New York: Penguin Books, 2013; Walrath, Dana, *Aliceheimers: Alzheimer's Through the Looking Glass,* Philadelphia: Penn State University Press, 2016.

6. Hume, Mary, "I Like Dancing and Singing and Prancing and Flinging: Using Poetry in Dementia Care," in Ann Burack-Weiss, Lynn Sara Lawrence, and Lynne Bamat Mijangos, eds., Foreword by Rita Charon, *Narrative in Social Work Practice: The Power and Possibility of Story,* New York: Columbia University Press, 2017: 144–155.

7. *Kazus Kukotskogo* was awarded the Russian Booker Prize in 2001 and was made into an acclaimed mini-series in 2005; *Still Alice* became a highly regarded motion picture in 2014. Throughout, I will refer to Ulitskaia's novel as *The Kukotsky Case;* Nemec Ignashev chose her title carefully, but I prefer my translation as it retains both the alliteration and the connection to Dostoevsky's *Crime and Punishment.*

8. Taylor, "On Recognition, Caring, and Dementia," 321.

9. For a longer, beautifully thoughtful meditation on these issues, see Solnit's 2013 *The Faraway Nearby*, in which the author explores her mother's dementia in similar terms: the power story exerts in living with Alzheimer's/dementia and for caregivers.

10. Taylor provides a chilling example of the effects of our cultural stories. She cites Sweeting and Gilhooly who interviewed caregivers of those with dementia. One man is a caregiver for his wife whom he describes as "a big baby" and who leaves her tied to the toilet when he needs to go out. Taylor also cites Kaufman's study of medical professionals who seem to think that a person with dementia is "as good as dead"; this belief then becomes a self-fulfilling prophecy, "On Recognition, Caring, and Dementia," 322–323.

11. Genova, Lisa, *Still Alice: A Novel,* New York: Pocket Books, 2007, 159.

12. Taylor, "On Recognition, Caring, and Dementia," 316, citing Fuchs, Elinor, *Making an Exit: A Mother-Daughter Drama with Alzheimer's, Machine Tools, and Laughter*, New York: Metropolitan Books, 2005, 4.

13. Taylor, "On Recognition, Caring, and Dementia," 316.

14. Genova, *Still Alice*, 126; 241.

15. Genova, *Still Alice*, 127. In Kali Quinn's play *Vamping*, there is a dementia test that illustrates the same point: the patient, Eleanor, wants to have a party (keep the cares together), but the medical professional conducting the test gives Eleanor demerit points for not sticking with the test—which, from Eleanor's point of view, is pointless. In this performance, Quinn beautifully points out the tyranny of such tests. The full citation is: *Vamping: Aging, Memory Loss & End-of-Life Ethics.* Performer: Kali Quinn. Duke University Medical Center, Durham, North Carolina. March 22, 2018. Solo Performance.

16. Genova, *Still Alice*, 241–248.
17. Genova, *Still Alice*, 248.
18. Genova, *Still Alice*, 235.
19. Genova, *Still Alice*, 292.
20. One reader of this essay, whose mother had dementia, noted that her mother would talk with great joy about people who had already died, experiencing them as present in her life again. This is a common experience of dementia, and mostly we take it as a sign that the patient is "dotty." What if we could experience a little of the joy of recovery with them?
21. It's a complicated story as the couple marries, believing that Elena's first husband is dead, and they then later discover that he died much later.
22. The Russian here is *vypadaiu.*
23. Ulitskaia, Liudmila, *Kazus Kukotskogo,* Moscow: EKSMO-Press, 2000. Translated by Diane Nemec Ignashev as *The Kutkotsky Enigma* and published by Northwestern University Press, 2016, 85.
24. Ulitskaia, *The Kukotsky Case*, 86.
25. The Russian here is *Vpala v sostoianie detstva . . . bessmyslenoi* (Russian text, 97).
26. Ulitskaia, *The Kukotsky Case*, 86.
27. Ulitskaia, *The Kukotsky Case*, 90.
28. Ulitskaia, *The Kukotsky Case*, 90.
29. Quotes are found in Ulitskaia, *The Kukotsky Case,* 93–95. "The middle world" in Russian is *Srednii mir* (Russian text, 108).
30. Throughout this essay, the "we" is a little complicated: by it, I mean the US certainly, but also those societies, mostly in the Global North, that are wealthy and medicalize dementia/Alzheimer's.
31. Ulitskaia, *The Kukotsky Case,* 129; 85.
32. Ulitskaia, *The Kukotsky Case*, 104–106. The Russian for the "Third Dimension" is *Tret'e sostoianie* (Russian text, 117–118).
33. The Russian is *vypadenie iz vneshnogo mira* (Russian text, 102).
34. Ulitskaia, *The Kukotsky Case,* 103.
35. Ulitskaia, *The Kukotsky Case,* 103.
36. Ulitskaia, *The Kukotsky Case,* 97.
37. Ulitskaia, *The Kukotsky Case*, 173.
38. Ulitskaia, *The Kukotsky Case,* 178.
39. Ulitskaia, *The Kukotsky Case,* 178.
40. Ulitskaia, *The Kukotsky Case,* 174.
41. The original Russian for the names "The Judean," "Skinhead," and Longhair is *Iudei, Britogolovyi,* and *Dlinnovolosyi,* respectively.
42. The Russian for this term is *Novenkaia*.
43. Ulitskaia, *The Kukotsky Case*, 173–174.
44. Ulitskaia, *The Kukotsky Case*, 174.
45. Ulitskaia, *The Kukotsky Case*, 191.
46. Ulitskaia, *The Kukotsky Case*, 209.
47. Ulitskaia, *The Kukotsky Case,* 196.

48. Ulitskaia, *The Kukotsky Case*, 220–221.

49. Pavel regains his name and identity through an encounter with Tolstoy (yes, that Tolstoy. The boundaries between fiction and reality are also unclear in this world, Ulitskaia, *The Kukotsky Case,* 227). In a literarily satisfying moment, Tolstoy shows up and discusses his mistakes in understanding (including that he now understands that carnal love is important for human beings, Ulitskaia, *The Kukotsky Case,* 237–242).

50. Ulitskaia, *The Kukotsky Case,* 232–234; 244–245. Elena's name begins to be used after Longhair plays the saxophone and after she is submersed in water. Water is very important to Elena throughout the novel. Her daughter Tanya and granddaughter Zhenya bathe her and it is in the water that Elena is most herself.

51. Ulitskaia, *The Kukotsky Case,* 392.

52. Ulitskaia, *The Kukotsky Case,* 393.

53. Power, *Dementia Beyond Drugs;* Taylor, "On Recognition, Caring, and Dementia"; Walrath, *Aliceheimer's: Alzheimer's Through the Looking Glass.*

54. In Avery Gordon's sense in *Ghostly Matters.* The whole book explicates her idea, but, briefly: "haunting describes how that which appears to be not there is often a seething presence, acting on and often meddling with taken-for-granted realities." Gordon, Avery, *Ghostly Matters*, Minneapolis: University of Minnesota Press, 1997, 8.

55. Research that shows how memory loss can be protective for those with trauma includes: Burri, Andrea, Andreas Maercker, Sandy Krammer, and Keti Simmen-Janevska, "Childhood Trauma and PTSD Symptoms Increase the Risk of Cognitive Impairment in a Sample of Former Indentured Child Laborers in Old Age," *PLoS One* 8(2), 2013; Greenberg, Mark S., Kaloyan Tanev, Marie-France Marin, and Roger K. Pitman, "Stress, PTSD, and Dementia," *Alzheimer's & Dementia* Vol 10: 3, Supplement, June 2014: S155–S165; Yaffe, Kristine, Eric Vittinghoff, Karla Lindquist, Deborah Barnes, Kenneth E. Covinsky, Thomas Neylan, Molly Kluse, and Charles Marmar, "Post-Traumatic Stress Disorder and Risk of Dementia among U.S. Veterans," *Arch Gen Psychiatry*, June 67.6 (2010): 608–613.

56. Ulitskaia, *The Kukotsky Case,* 414–415.

57. I recognize that it is a bit awkward to cite Russian literature in an essay that is about an American and a Russian novel. Although of course my imagination is shaped by other literature as well, it is Russian literature in which I have lived deeply for more than 25 years, so it deserves a special recognition—especially because Russian literature is so often left out of discussions of world literature.

WORKS CITED

Applewhite, Ashton. *This Chair Rocks: A Manifesto against Ageism.* Self-published by Networked Books, 2016.

Burri, Andrea, Andreas Maercker, Sandy Krammer, and Keti Simmen-Janevska. "Childhood Trauma and PTSD Symptoms Increase the Risk of Cognitive Impairment in a Sample of Former Indentured Child Laborers in Old Age." *PLoS One* 8(2), 2013.

Fuchs, Elinor. *Making an Exit: A Mother-Daughter Drama with Alzheimer's, Machine Tools, and Laughter*. New York: Metropolitan Books, 2005.

Genova, Lisa. *Still Alice: A Novel.* New York: Pocket Books, 2007.

Goscilo, Helena. *Dehexing Sex: Russian Womanhood during and after Glasnost.* Ann Arbor: University of Michigan Press, 1996.

Gordon, Avery. *Ghostly Matters*. Minneapolis: University of Minnesota Press, 1997.

Greenberg, Mark S., Kaloyan Tanev, Marie-France Marin, and Roger K. Pitman. "Stress, PTSD, and Dementia." *Alzheimer's & Dementia* Vol 10: 3, Supplement, June 2014: S155–S165.

Hume, Mary. "I Like Dancing and Singing and Prancing and Flinging: Using Poetry in Dementia Care," in Ann Burack-Weiss, Lynn Sara Lawrence, and Lynne Bamat Mijangos, eds., Foreword by Rita Charon, *Narrative in Social Work Practice: The Power and Possibility of Story.* New York: Columbia University Press, 2017: 144–155.

Power, G. Allen. *Dementia beyond Drugs: Changing the Culture of Care.* 2d edn. Baltimore, MD: Health Professions Press, Inc, 2017.

Skomp, Elizabeth and Benjamin Sutcliffe. *Ludmila Ulitskaya and the Art of Tolerance.* Madison, Wisconsin: University of Wisconsin Press, 2015.

Solnit, Rebecca. *The Faraway Nearby.* New York: Penguin Books, 2013.

Taylor, Janelle S. "On Recognition, Caring, and Dementia." *Medical Anthropology Quarterly* 22.4 (2008): 313–335.

Ulitskaia, Liudmila. *Kazus Kukotskogo.* Moscow: EKSMO-Press, 2000. Translated by Diane Nemec Ignashev as *The Kutkotsky Enigma* and published by Northwestern University Press, 2016.

Walrath, Dana. *Aliceheimers: Alzheimer's Through the Looking Glass.* Philadelphia: Penn State University Press, 2016.

Yaffe, Kristine, Eric Vittinghoff, Karla Lindquist, Deborah Barnes, Kenneth E. Covinsky, Thomas Neylan, Molly Kluse, and Charles Marmar. "Post-Traumatic Stress Disorder and Risk of Dementia among U.S. Veterans." *Arch Gen Psychiatry,* June 67.6 (2010): 608–613.

Index

Page references for figures are italicized.

About the Contributors

Angela Brintlinger, PhD, is Professor and Chair of Graduate Studies at the Department of Slavic and East European Languages and Cultures, as well as the Director of the Center for Slavic and East European Studies, at The Ohio State University. She is the author of *Writing a Usable Past: Russian Literary Culture, 1917–1937* (2008) and *Chapaev and His Comrades: War and the Russian Literary Hero Across the Twentieth Century* (2012). She is the co-editor with Ilya Vinitsky of *Madness and the Mad in Russian Culture* (2007) and the co-editor with Carol Apollonio of *Chekhov for the 21st Century* (2013).

Jehanne Gheith, MSW, LCSW, PhDm is a Licensed Clinical Social Worker and a tenured professor at Duke. She works at Duke Hospice as a clinical social worker and as a grief counselor and has a private practice specializing in grief counseling, including pet loss, aging, illness, and wellness transitions. As a professor, she teaches courses on Russian culture and on Medical Ethics, Aging, and End of Life Care; one of these courses is a Service Learning course and students volunteered with Duke Hospice and at the VA Hospice. In both her academic publications and her clinical work, her focus is on narrative and loss.

Maria P. Kuzybaeva, PhD, is a historian and independent scholar with a specialty in medical museum studies. She worked as a Chief Curator of the Medical Museum at the Russian Academy of Medical Sciences (RAMS) (1995–2000), a senior researcher at the RAMS Scientific Association (Medical Encyclopedia) and the RAMS Institute of the History of Medicine (2001–2013), and a senior researcher at the National Research Institute of Public Health named after N.A. Semashko (2013–2016). She is the author of more than 700 publications on the history of medical museums in the Russian Empire and in the Russian Federation.

Irina Markovina is Director of the Institute of Linguistics and Intercultural Communication at Sechenov University (Sechenov First Moscow State Medical University). She is a representative of the Russian School of Psycholinguistics, a member of the editorial board of the peer-reviewed Russian journal *Problems of Psycholinguistics*, as well as a reviewer for *MedEdPublish* (AMEE). She has published over 200 works including research articles, books, textbooks, and medical dictionaries. She also teaches courses in English for Medical Purposes, Medical Translation, and Ethno-psycholinguistics, as well as conducts research in these fields, thus promoting intercultural communication and international cooperation.

As leader of the international staff at Sechenov University, she is actively involved in developing the English language environment at both Sechenov and other medical universities.

Jonathan McFarland is Director of the Academic Writing Office at Sechenov University in Moscow. Jonathan does research in Discourse Analysis, Sociolinguistics, and Composition Studies. He is President of the Doctor as Humanist Program (Palma de Mayorca, 2017–present) and Associate Professor in the Faculty of Medicine at Universidad Autonoma Madrid. He is a member of the Moscow Office Committee, ASME (Association for the Study of Medical Education, a Committee member of EUNAMES (European Narrative Medicine Society), and of ASOMEGA (Association of Galician Doctors).

When not working, he enjoys living the quiet life in Soller, in the beautiful Tramuntana mountains, enjoying gardening and walking in the mountains with his family.

Melissa L. Miller, PhD, is Assistant Teaching Professor and Director of Undergraduate Studies in Russian at the University of Notre Dame. She also teaches in the Medicine and the Liberal Arts program in the Reilly Center for Science, Technology, and Values at the University of Notre Dame. Her articles have appeared in *The Russian Review* and *The Slavic and East European Journal*. Her research interests include the medical humanities, science fiction in Russia and Eastern Europe, gender studies, and Second Language Acquisition.

Evgeniya L. Panova, PhD, is Head of the History of Medicine Department at the Medical Institute at Peoples' Friendship University of Russia (RUDN

University), Moscow. Her work focuses on History of Medicine, Bioethics, History of Russian Neurology, Philosophy of Medicine and Medical Humanities. She has taught courses in bioethics, the history of medicine, the history of Russian surgery, and the history of pharmacy at the Department of Medical Humanities at Sechenov First Moscow State Medical University. She has received an award for the development of research work with students from the Russian Society for the History of Medicine (2016).

Konstantin Starikov, PhD, MLIS, is an independent scholar and librarian. He worked as Head of Access Services at Alumni Medical Library, Boston University, from 2008–2020. He served as a member of the ASEEES CLIR Committee on Education and Access, 2017–2021, and as a Slavic Digital Humanities Officer for Slavic DH, ASEEES (Association for Slavic, Eastern European, & Eurasian Studies), 2016–2017.

Maria S. Tutorskaya is a Senior Researcher at the Russian Medical Museum, FSSBI (N.A. Semashko National Research Institute of Public Health), Moscow, Russian Federation. A medical historian, Maria's research interests center on social history, art history, medicine and literature, and the history of medical museums.

Maria is a member of the Museum Alumni Organizing Committee at the Pushkin State Museum of Fine Arts and the founder of the Medical Humanities Online Seminar Series "Corona Talks." Maria is a graduate of the Faculty of History at Moscow State University and the Department of Ethnology in 2004. In 2009, she graduated from the Moscow College as a nurse. She worked as a Senior Lecturer at the History of Medicine, Bioethics, National History and Culturology Department of Sechenov University (2006–2016).

Natalia Vygovskaia holds the degree of Candidate of Philological Sciences from Moscow State University. Her dissertation explored Chechen veterans' post-war narratives (1990–2000). Currently, she is a PhD Candidate in the Department of Slavic Studies at Brown University. Her research focuses on medical ethics in Russian culture in the late nineteenth through the twentieth centuries. Her dissertation traces the cultural history of medical ethics in the journal *Vrach* (*The Physician*), doctors' memoirs, and Russian literature (1880–1910). Natalia's other research interests include scientific biography, heroic narratives, geocriticism, and poetry translation. She is an administrator and chief editor of the online journal of poetry translation "Purple Ink," hosted by Brown University.

Frederick H. White, PhD, is Professor of Russian and Integrated Studies in the Department of Integrated Studies. He is one of the leading specialists on the Russian writer Leonid Andreev and has published in the areas of Russian Modernism, psychiatry, and literature in the Russian fin de siècle, the economics of culture, and post-Soviet cinema.

www.ingramcontent.com/pod-product-compliance
Lightning Source LLC
Chambersburg PA
CBHW071251180926
51613CB00001B/13
* 9 7 8 1 4 9 8 5 9 2 1 5 4 *